JEANNE HOUSTON

Borderline Personality Disorder: A Woman's Perspective

Contents

1

Introduction and Personal Context

Borderline Personality Disorder (BPD) is a complex and often misunderstood mental health condition. This book is born out of both personal experience and rigorous research, designed to offer a compassionate guide for managing BPD from a woman's perspective. In this introductory chapter, I aim to lay the groundwork by sharing my own journey, discussing why I felt compelled to write about this subject, and outlining the structure of the book. Along the way, I will reference established works in the field to provide readers with a broader context and additional resources for further exploration.

Personal Journey and the Spark for Writing

My journey with BPD has been one marked by moments of profound insight, overwhelming despair, and, ultimately, a gradual realization of self-compassion and resilience. Growing up, I often felt like I was walking on a tightrope—oscillating between extremes of emotion and struggling to reconcile my inner world with societal expectations. The isolation I experienced was

1

compounded by the stigma that often surrounds mental health, particularly conditions like BPD.

I vividly remember the turning point when I finally accepted my diagnosis. It wasn't a moment of defeat but rather an opening of a new chapter—one where I began to understand that my struggles were not a personal failing but rather a part of a larger tapestry of mental health challenges that many women face. This realization was both liberating and daunting. I began to delve into literature and research, seeking to understand the neurobiology, psychology, and sociocultural factors contributing to my experiences. Books such as Marsha Linehan's *Cognitive-Behavioral Treatment of Borderline Personality Disorder* provided not only validation but also practical strategies that helped me begin to regain control over my life.

The Intersection of Research and Personal Narrative

This book is structured around the idea that true understanding comes from the intersection of empirical research and lived experience. As you read these pages, you will encounter a blend of scientific insight and personal narrative. I have drawn upon case studies, interviews with mental health professionals, and established research to create a comprehensive resource that is both informative and empathetic.

For instance, works like *I Hate You, Don't Leave Me* by Jerold J. Kreisman and Hal Straus have been influential in shaping public perceptions of BPD. Although controversial at times, this book opened the door for many to see the human side of the disorder, a perspective I hope to echo here. Similarly, *Stop Walking on Eggshells* by Paul Mason and Randi Kreger has provided valuable strategies for managing relationships affected by BPD, highlighting the need for healthy boundaries and communication. By referencing such seminal works, I aim to build a bridge between the established literature and the personal experiences that drive my advocacy.

What Readers Can Expect

Throughout this book, the chapters will guide you through various aspects of BPD—from understanding the clinical and neurological underpinnings of the disorder to exploring the impact of trauma, emotional dysregulation, and the importance of building a supportive community. Each chapter is designed to stand alone as a valuable resource, yet together they form a coherent narrative that speaks to both the science and the soul of living with BPD.

The journey begins with understanding the basics of BPD—its symptoms, the diagnostic process, and the unique ways in which it affects women. This is crucial because the experience of BPD is not monolithic. The emotional intensity, relationship challenges, and identity struggles often manifest differently in women compared to men. Societal expectations and gender roles further complicate these experiences, a nuance that I will explore in depth throughout the book.

In the subsequent chapters, we will delve into the biology of BPD, examining research that highlights how factors such as brain structure and neurotransmitter imbalances contribute to the disorder. The inclusion of case studies, drawn from both my personal encounters and the experiences of others, will provide a human face to these scientific findings. For example, research and personal accounts described in *The Buddha and the Borderline* by Kiera Van Gelder illustrate how integrating therapeutic practices like Dialectical Behavior Therapy (DBT) can lead to transformative change.

The Role of Research in Shaping Our Understanding

The importance of research in demystifying BPD cannot be overstated. Over the past few decades, advances in psychology and neuroscience have provided critical insights into how the brain processes emotion and stress. Studies have shown that individuals with BPD often experience heightened emotional sensitivity and slower return to emotional baseline after intense experiences. These scientific observations help explain the seemingly erratic behavior and intense emotional responses that are characteristic of the disorder.

Moreover, research has highlighted the significant role that early life experiences play in the development of BPD. Trauma, especially in the formative years, has been identified as a key factor that can predispose individuals to developing the disorder. Understanding this link is crucial for both prevention and treatment. In this book, I integrate findings from longitudinal studies and meta-analyses that reveal how early trauma not only affects emotional regulation but also shapes the trajectory of personal relationships and self-identity.

One of the most influential frameworks I encountered was provided by Marsha Linehan's work on DBT. Her book has served as a cornerstone for understanding how structured therapeutic interventions can equip individuals with the skills necessary to manage emotional turmoil. By referencing such research, I hope to empower readers with evidence-based techniques that have proven effective for many in similar situations.

The Feminine Perspective on BPD

Focusing on the feminine perspective, this book acknowledges that women often face unique challenges when dealing with BPD. Societal pressures related to appearance, behavior, and emotional expression can exacerbate the symptoms of BPD. Women are frequently expected to maintain calm and composed exteriors, even when internal chaos reigns. This dissonance between societal expectations and internal reality can lead to feelings of inadequacy and further destabilize emotional well-being.

Books like *Women Who Run with the Wolves* by Clarissa Pinkola Estés have long explored the deep, archetypal forces that shape women's lives. Although not exclusively about BPD, such works provide a rich tapestry of insights into the emotional and psychological experiences that many women share. Integrating these perspectives helps illuminate why traditional therapeutic models might need adaptation to better serve women with BPD.

This narrative is not merely about the struggle but also about reclaiming one's identity and power. Each chapter of this book will illustrate how, through self-discovery and the right therapeutic interventions, women can transform the challenges of BPD into avenues for growth. The goal is not only to manage the disorder but also to celebrate the resilience and strength that often lie hidden beneath the surface of emotional turmoil.

Laying the Groundwork for Future Chapters

As we embark on this journey together, it's important to recognize that this book is both a guide and a conversation. It is written in the hope of providing comfort and clarity to those who see parts of their own stories reflected in these pages. Whether you are newly diagnosed, have been living with BPD for years, or support someone who is, the insights contained herein are meant to offer both validation and practical strategies.

The chapters that follow will delve into specific aspects of BPD:

- **Understanding BPD from a Clinical Standpoint:** We will examine the diagnostic criteria, explore how BPD manifests uniquely in women, and debunk common myths.
- **Exploring the Neurobiological and Psychological Foundations:** Here, we will discuss the latest research on brain function, genetic predispositions, and the psychological theories that shed light on the disorder.
- **The Impact of Trauma and Emotional Dysregulation:** A detailed look at how early life experiences and trauma contribute to BPD, supported by both research and compelling case studies.
- **Therapeutic Journeys and Recovery:** Real-life case studies will illustrate diverse paths to healing, offering insights into how different therapeutic modalities—including DBT, Cognitive Behavioral Therapy (CBT), and emerging treatments—can be applied.
- **Building Support Systems and Embracing Self-Care:** This section will focus on the importance of social support, setting healthy boundaries, and incorporating self-care and mindfulness practices into daily life.

Throughout these chapters, I will continue to weave in references to seminal works and recent studies that have shaped our understanding of BPD. Books such as *I Hate You, Don't Leave Me* and *Stop Walking on Eggshells* have provided both inspiration and practical advice that continues to influence the discourse around this complex disorder.

Final Thoughts

The intent of this book is not to offer a one-size-fits-all solution. BPD, like any mental health condition, is multifaceted, and the path to managing it is deeply personal. However, by grounding our discussion in both research and real-life experiences, I hope to create a resource that is as empathetic as it is informative.

As you continue reading, remember that you are not alone in this journey. Whether you are experiencing BPD firsthand or supporting someone who is, the challenges you face are acknowledged and validated. Together, we will explore the intricacies of BPD, drawing on both the latest scientific research and the powerful narratives of women who have walked this path before you.

In the pages that follow, I invite you to embark on a journey of discovery, healing, and empowerment. May this book serve as a beacon of hope, illuminating the way towards a more balanced, resilient, and compassionate future.

By integrating personal insights with established research and referencing influential books in the field, this chapter lays a solid foundation for understanding BPD from a woman's perspective. It sets the stage for a deep dive into both the scientific and personal dimensions of the disorder—a journey that is as much about understanding oneself as it is about embracing the possibility of healing.

2

Understanding BPD – Clinical and Personal Perspectives

Borderline Personality Disorder (BPD) is a multifaceted and often misunderstood condition that challenges both clinical definitions and everyday perceptions. In this chapter, we delve into the clinical aspects of BPD while intertwining personal narratives that highlight its profound impact on women. We will explore diagnostic criteria, symptomatology, and the unique ways in which BPD manifests in women, drawing upon seminal texts and recent research to illuminate both scientific and lived experiences.

Defining BPD: The Clinical Landscape

BPD is characterized by pervasive instability in moods, behavior, self-image, and functioning. Clinically, the Diagnostic and Statistical Manual of Mental Disorders (DSM-5) defines BPD through a series of criteria including fear of abandonment, intense interpersonal relationships, chronic feelings of emptiness, and impulsive behaviors. These diagnostic guidelines provide a structure for understanding the disorder but often fall short of capturing its emotional depth and complexity.

Books such as *I Hate You, Don't Leave Me* by Jerold J. Kreisman and Hal Straus have played a pivotal role in translating these clinical criteria into real-world experiences. Kreisman and Straus present a compassionate yet stark view of BPD, showing how the disorder can disrupt every facet of a person's life, from work to personal relationships. Their work underscores that while clinical definitions offer a starting point, the emotional turmoil and identity struggles inherent in BPD require a more nuanced exploration.

Diagnostic Criteria and Beyond

The DSM-5 criteria for BPD include:

· **Frantic efforts to avoid real or imagined abandonment.**
· **A pattern of unstable and intense interpersonal relationships.**
· **Identity disturbance.**
· **Impulsivity in at least two areas that are potentially self-damaging.**
· **Recurrent suicidal behavior, gestures, or threats.**
· **Affective instability due to marked reactivity of mood.**
· **Chronic feelings of emptiness.**
· **Inappropriate, intense anger or difficulty controlling anger.**
· **Transient, stress-related paranoid ideation or severe dissociative symptoms.**

These criteria provide a clinical framework that helps mental health professionals diagnose and treat BPD. However, many individuals—especially women—experience these symptoms in ways that are deeply personal and contextually bound. In her groundbreaking work, *Stop Walking on Eggshells* by Paul Mason and Randi Kreger, the authors explore how these clinical symptoms manifest in day-to-day interactions and relationships, offering insights into the emotional and relational dynamics that are often overshadowed by a purely diagnostic approach.

The Unique Experience of Women with BPD

While BPD affects individuals regardless of gender, the experience of the disorder in women often carries distinct nuances. Societal expectations and cultural pressures can exacerbate the symptoms of BPD in women, making the path to diagnosis and treatment uniquely challenging. Women are frequently socialized to be nurturing, emotionally expressive, and self-sacrificing—a combination that can intensify the internal conflict when faced with the instability of BPD.

Societal Influences and Gender Roles

The societal script for women often emphasizes stability, empathy, and calmness. When women experience the intense emotional fluctuations characteristic of BPD, these cultural expectations can lead to feelings of inadequacy and shame. In *Women Who Run with the Wolves* by Clarissa Pinkola Estés, the narrative delves into the archetypal patterns that shape a woman's life, suggesting that the inner wildness and emotional depth inherent in many women are not only natural but necessary. However, when these traits are labeled as symptoms of a disorder, the very essence of what it means to be a woman can be misunderstood and pathologized.

This misinterpretation can be seen in the way society often views emotional intensity in women. Rather than being cel‐ ebrated as a sign of passion or creativity, intense emotional expression is frequently stigmatized. The resulting internal conflict can deepen the emotional dysregulation experienced by those with BPD, making it crucial to consider the gendered dimensions of the disorder. This perspective is supported by research indicating that women are more likely to be diagnosed with BPD than men—a discrepancy that might partly reflect the interplay between societal norms and clinical practices.

The Lived Experience: Narratives and Case Studies

Personal narratives and case studies offer a window into the lived experience of BPD that clinical descriptions alone cannot provide. For example, consider the story of Sarah—a composite case study drawn from multiple clinical accounts and personal interviews. Sarah's narrative is marked by a recurring fear of abandonment, which not only strained her relationships but also undermined her sense of self‐worth. Her experiences resonate with the descriptions found in *I Hate You, Don't Leave Me*, where the emotional volatility and relational turbulence of BPD are depicted with raw honesty.

Sarah's journey illustrates a common theme: the struggle to reconcile internal emotional chaos with external expectations. Like many women with BPD, Sarah was caught in a relentless cycle of idealizing and devaluing those closest to her. The intense highs and lows of her interpersonal relationships were compounded by the societal pressure to remain composed and resilient. Such stories, when viewed alongside clinical research, reveal the multifaceted nature of BPD—a condition that is as much about external relationships as it is about inner turmoil.

Bridging Clinical Research and Personal Narratives

One of the central aims of this book is to bridge the gap between clinical research and the personal experiences of those living with BPD. While research provides critical insights into the mechanisms underlying the disorder, personal narratives bring to light the human aspects that data alone cannot capture.

Integrating Research Findings

Recent studies in neuroscience and psychology have shed light on the underlying mechanisms of BPD. For instance, neuroimaging research has revealed differences in brain structure and function, particularly in regions involved in emotion regulation and impulse control. These findings suggest that the heightened emotional sensitivity observed in BPD may have a biological basis. Works like *The Buddha and the Borderline* by Kiera Van Gelder highlight how these scientific discoveries can be integrated into therapeutic practices such as Dialectical Behavior Therapy (DBT), providing patients with tools to manage their emotional responses.

Research also points to the impact of early childhood trauma on the development of BPD. Longitudinal studies have consistently shown that individuals with a history of childhood abuse or neglect are at a higher risk of developing BPD later in life. This connection underscores the importance of trauma-informed care and the need for therapeutic interventions that address both the psychological and physiological aspects of the disorder. By examining these studies alongside personal accounts, we begin to see a more complete picture of how early experiences shape the trajectory of BPD.

The Role of Therapy and Self-Discovery

Therapeutic interventions are central to managing BPD, and many women have found solace in approaches that combine both clinical techniques and personal insight. DBT, a form of therapy developed specifically for BPD, emphasizes mindfulness, distress tolerance, emotion regulation, and interpersonal effectiveness. Marsha Linehan's work on DBT has been transformative, providing a structured framework that empowers patients to navigate the emotional storms of BPD.

Books like *Cognitive-Behavioral Treatment of Borderline Personality Disorder* by Marsha Linehan not only outline therapeutic techniques but also provide evidence of their effectiveness. These resources have been instrumental in shaping modern approaches to treating BPD and offer hope to those who feel overwhelmed by the disorder. Through a combination of research-backed strategies and individual effort, many women have successfully redefined their relationship with their emotions, moving from a place of reactivity to one of mindful awareness and resilience.

The Complex Interplay of Identity and Emotion

A defining feature of BPD is the struggle with identity. For many women, this battle is not just about managing emotions but also about forging a sense of self that feels authentic in a world that often imposes restrictive roles. The internal conflict of wanting to be both strong and vulnerable, independent and connected, is a recurring theme in the lives of those with BPD.

Identity Disturbance in BPD

Identity disturbance—a core symptom of BPD—is characterized by a markedly unstable self-image or sense of self. This instability can manifest in various ways, from frequent shifts in personal goals and values to a profound uncertainty about one's place in the world. The literature on BPD often highlights how this lack of a stable identity can lead to impulsivity and erratic decision-making, further complicating the lives of those affected.

In *Stop Walking on Eggshells*, Mason and Kreger emphasize that understanding and accepting one's identity is a critical component of managing BPD. The process of self-discovery is both painful and liberating, requiring individuals to confront deeply ingrained fears of rejection and abandonment. For many women, the journey toward a coherent sense of self involves reconciling internal conflicts between societal expectations and personal desires. This journey is marked by setbacks and triumphs alike, forming the basis for many of the case studies and personal narratives presented throughout this book.

Emotional Intensity and Its Dual Nature

The emotional intensity experienced by those with BPD is often described as a double-edged sword. On one hand, the depth of emotion can lead to creative expression, empathy, and passion; on the other, it can result in overwhelming distress and self-destructive behavior. This dual nature is central to understanding BPD—it is not merely a disorder to be eliminated, but a complex human experience that demands compassion and insight.

The writings of Clarissa Pinkola Estés in *Women Who Run with the Wolves* resonate here, as they celebrate the raw, untamed aspects of the feminine spirit. Estés' work encourages women to embrace their inner wildness rather than suppress it, suggesting that what is often labeled as a disorder may also be a misunderstood strength. Recognizing this duality is crucial for anyone seeking to manage BPD: it involves harnessing the creative potential of intense emotion while developing strategies to mitigate its disruptive effects.

Towards a Holistic Understanding

A holistic approach to understanding BPD must account for both the clinical and personal dimensions of the disorder. This chapter has attempted to lay the groundwork by defining BPD from a clinical standpoint, exploring the gender-specific challenges faced by women, and bridging these aspects with personal narratives and research findings. As we move forward in this book, it is essential to remember that each story of BPD is unique. No single definition or clinical framework can fully encompass the lived reality of those struggling with this condition.

By combining insights from authoritative texts like *I Hate You, Don't Leave Me*, *Stop Walking on Eggshells*, and *The Buddha and the Borderline* with real-life experiences, we can develop a richer, more empathetic understanding of BPD. This integration not only enhances our clinical knowledge but also validates

15

the personal journeys of countless women who navigate the turbulent waters of BPD every day.

Conclusion

Understanding BPD requires more than a list of symptoms or a clinical diagnosis—it demands an appreciation of the interplay between biology, personal history, societal expectations, and the profound quest for identity. Women with BPD often face the added burden of societal judgment, making their journey toward self-acceptance and emotional balance even more challenging. Yet, within this struggle lies an opportunity for profound transformation—a chance to reclaim one's identity and harness the intense emotions that characterize the disorder.

In the chapters ahead, we will continue to explore the myriad facets of BPD—from the neurobiological underpinnings and the impact of trauma to the transformative power of therapy and self-care. Each chapter will build upon the foundation laid here, offering insights that are both scientifically grounded and deeply personal. My hope is that by understanding the clinical and personal perspectives of BPD, readers will be better equipped to navigate their own journeys, find effective treatment strategies, and ultimately, embrace the possibility of healing.

As we close this chapter, I invite you to reflect on your own experiences or those of the women you care about. Recognize that the struggle with BPD is not a solitary one; it is a shared journey of discovery, resilience, and, ultimately, empowerment. The road ahead is not without its challenges, but it is also filled with the promise of growth and transformation—a promise that we will explore in depth in the coming chapters.

By weaving together clinical definitions, societal observations, and personal narratives, this chapter has aimed to provide a comprehensive understanding of BPD from both a scientific and a deeply human perspective. It is through this dual lens that we can begin to appreciate the complexity of BPD and the unique challenges it presents for women. The references to influential works such as *I Hate You, Don't Leave Me*, *Stop Walking on Eggshells*, and *Women Who Run with the Wolves* serve not only as a foundation for our discussion but also as a reminder of the rich tapestry of literature that has helped shape our understanding of this intricate disorder.

In the next chapter, we will turn our focus to the science behind BPD, delving into the neurological and psychological research that explains why the disorder manifests the way it does. This exploration will provide further insight into how biological predispositions and early life experiences converge to shape the lived experience of BPD, ultimately equipping readers with the knowledge needed to approach treatment and self-care from an informed and empowered perspective.

3

The Science Behind BPD – Neurology and Psychology

Borderline Personality Disorder (BPD) is not solely a matter of emotions and personal history—it is also a condition deeply rooted in the biological and psychological fabric of the human brain. In this chapter, we delve into the science behind BPD, exploring the neurological and psychological research that helps explain why the disorder manifests in such complex ways. We will examine how brain structure, neurotransmitter systems, genetic predispositions, and psychological theories converge to create the symptoms and behaviors characteristic of BPD. Drawing on seminal texts and the latest research, this chapter aims to provide a comprehensive scientific foundation to support both clinical understanding and personal insights.

Neurological Foundations of BPD

Brain Structure and Function

Recent advances in neuroimaging have significantly improved our understanding of BPD. Studies have consistently shown that individuals with BPD exhibit differences in the structure and function of several key brain regions. For example, the amygdala—a region involved in processing emotions—tends to be hyperactive in people with BPD. This heightened activity may explain why emotions are experienced so intensely and why individuals with BPD often struggle to regulate their feelings. Additionally, research has pointed to alterations in the prefrontal cortex, the brain area responsible for impulse control and executive functioning. These neural differences can help explain the impulsivity and erratic decision-making often observed in BPD.

Marsha Linehan's groundbreaking work on Dialectical Behavior Therapy (DBT) is deeply intertwined with these findings. In *Cognitive-Behavioral Treatment of Borderline Personality Disorder*, Linehan not only introduces practical strategies for managing emotional dysregulation but also alludes to the neurobiological underpinnings that make these strategies effective. By focusing on mindfulness and distress tolerance, DBT can help compensate for the reduced regulatory control exerted by the prefrontal cortex.

Neurotransmitter Systems and Genetic Influences

Beyond structural differences, neurotransmitter imbalances have also been implicated in BPD. Neurotransmitters such as serotonin, dopamine, and norepinephrine play crucial roles in mood regulation and emotional responses. Abnormalities in these chemical messengers can lead to the heightened sensitivity and rapid mood shifts characteristic of BPD. Although research in this area is ongoing, current studies suggest that a combination of genetic factors and environmental stressors can disrupt neurotransmitter functioning, thereby contributing to the disorder.

Genetics also plays a significant role in the predisposition to BPD. Family studies have shown that BPD tends to run in families, suggesting a hereditary component. However, genetic vulnerability is not destiny. Environmental factors—especially early childhood trauma—can interact with genetic predispositions to trigger the onset of BPD. This gene-environment interplay underscores the importance of adopting both a biological and psychosocial perspective when examining the disorder.

Psychological Theories Explaining BPD

Attachment Theory and Early Relationships

One of the most influential psychological frameworks for understanding BPD is attachment theory. This theory, originally developed by John Bowlby and further expanded by Mary Ainsworth, posits that the quality of early relationships with caregivers significantly influences emotional development and future relational patterns. In individuals with BPD, disrupted or insecure attachment experiences are common. These early experiences can lead to an overwhelming fear of abandonment and difficulties in establishing stable, trusting relationships.

Books such as *I Hate You, Don't Leave Me* by Jerold J. Kreisman and Hal Straus vividly describe how attachment issues manifest in BPD. The text illustrates how early disruptions in caregiver relationships can create a template for future interpersonal interactions—one marked by oscillations between idealization and devaluation. This fluctuating dynamic often leaves those with BPD in a perpetual state of emotional turmoil, continuously seeking validation while simultaneously fearing rejection.

Emotion Dysregulation and Cognitive Distortions

Another psychological perspective central to understanding BPD is the concept of emotion dysregulation. Emotion dysregulation refers to difficulties in managing and responding to emotional experiences in an adaptive manner. Individuals with BPD often experience emotions that are not only more intense but also longer-lasting than those of people without the disorder. This persistent emotional reactivity is frequently accompanied by cognitive distortions—patterns of thinking that are overly negative or self-critical.

In *The Buddha and the Borderline* by Kiera Van Gelder, the author explores how integrating mindfulness practices can help moderate these intense emotions. The book provides insights into how mindfulness-based strategies encourage individuals to observe their emotions without judgment, thereby reducing the likelihood of cognitive distortions spiraling into crisis. By combining mindfulness with cognitive-behavioral techniques, many have found a pathway toward achieving greater emotional balance—a goal that resonates with both scientific findings and personal experiences.

The Role of Trauma in Shaping the Psyche

Trauma, particularly in early childhood, is a recurrent theme in the psychological literature on BPD. Traumatic experiences such as abuse, neglect, or the sudden loss of a caregiver can significantly disrupt the normal development of emotional regulation. The resulting scars often manifest as chronic feelings of emptiness, impulsivity, and unstable relationships— hallmarks of BPD.

Trauma theory suggests that these early adverse experiences can fundamentally alter one's cognitive and emotional processing. For many women with BPD, the trauma of their past is intricately woven into their present struggles with identity and emotional stability. In *Stop Walking on Eggshells* by Paul Mason and Randi Kreger, the discussion often revolves around how unaddressed trauma not only exacerbates the symptoms of BPD but also complicates the process of establishing healthy interpersonal relationships. This perspective reinforces the need for trauma-informed care, where both the biological and psychological impacts of early trauma are addressed through integrated therapeutic approaches.

Bridging Neurology and Psychology: An Integrated Model

The Interplay of Brain and Behavior

The convergence of neurological and psychological research offers a more holistic view of BPD. On one hand, neuroimaging and biochemical studies provide tangible evidence of the physical changes in the brain associated with BPD. On the other, psychological theories and case studies illuminate how these changes translate into the lived experience of emotional instability and interpersonal challenges.

Consider the case of Emily, a composite character drawn from numerous clinical accounts and research interviews. Emily's brain imaging results revealed hyperactivity in the amygdala and reduced activity in her prefrontal cortex—findings that correlate closely with her reported experiences of intense emotional responses and impulsive decisions. Simultaneously, her personal narrative highlighted long-standing issues with attachment, stemming from an unpredictable childhood marked by inconsistent caregiving. Emily's story is a powerful example of how biological predispositions and psychological factors intertwine, creating a complex web of challenges that require multifaceted treatment approaches.

Therapeutic Implications of an Integrated Approach

Understanding the scientific underpinnings of BPD is not an end in itself—it serves as a foundation for developing effective treatment strategies. An integrated approach that addresses both the neurological and psychological aspects of BPD is essential for fostering lasting recovery.

Dialectical Behavior Therapy (DBT) is a prime example of such an integrated approach. DBT combines cognitive-behavioral techniques with mindfulness practices, directly targeting the dysregulation of emotions while also addressing the cognitive distortions that exacerbate interpersonal conflicts. Marsha Linehan's seminal work in developing DBT, as outlined in *Cognitive-Behavioral Treatment of Borderline Personality Disorder*, has been pivotal in demonstrating how therapeutic interventions can be tailored to counteract both the biological vulnerabilities and the psychological traumas inherent in BPD.

Moreover, emerging research on pharmacological treatments offers additional support for an integrated model. While no medication can "cure" BPD, certain drugs—such as selective serotonin reuptake inhibitors (SSRIs) or mood stabilizers—can help manage specific symptoms by addressing the neurochemical imbalances in the brain. When combined with psychotherapy, these medications can significantly improve the quality of life for many individuals with BPD.

The Future of BPD Research

The field of BPD research is continuously evolving. Advances in genetic studies, neuroimaging, and psychopharmacology are likely to deepen our understanding of the disorder in the coming years. Future research may reveal more about the interplay between genetic predispositions and environmental triggers, potentially paving the way for personalized treatment strategies. These developments hold the promise of not only enhancing the effectiveness of current therapies but also providing new insights into preventive measures.

Books like *The Buddha and the Borderline* and *I Hate You, Don't Leave Me* serve as both historical landmarks and ongoing inspirations in this area. They remind us that the journey toward understanding BPD is one of constant discovery—a journey where science and personal narrative inform and enrich each other.

Integrating Science with Personal Experience

A major aim of this book is to demystify BPD by linking scientific research with the personal experiences of women who live with the disorder. For many, understanding the biological and psychological mechanisms behind their symptoms can be both enlightening and empowering. It provides a framework to make sense of what might otherwise feel like random, uncontrollable emotional upheavals.

For example, when a woman with BPD experiences an intense emotional response, understanding that her brain may be predisposed to hyperactivity in the amygdala offers a sense of relief. It shifts the narrative from one of personal failure to one that acknowledges the inherent challenges posed by the disorder. This perspective is crucial not only for self-compassion but also for fostering a collaborative relationship with mental health professionals who can tailor treatment to address both neurobiological and psychological needs.

Conclusion

In this chapter, we have explored the scientific landscape of BPD through the lenses of neurology and psychology. By examining the structural and functional changes in the brain, the role of neurotransmitters, genetic influences, and psychological theories such as attachment and trauma, we have constructed a comprehensive picture of the disorder. The integration of these diverse strands of research underscores that BPD is not a singularly defined condition—it is a complex interplay of biology, psychology, and environment.

References to seminal works such as Marsha Linehan's

Cognitive-Behavioral Treatment of Borderline Personality Disorder, Jerold J. Kreisman and Hal Straus's *I Hate You, Don't Leave Me*, and Clarissa Pinkola Estés' *Women Who Run with the Wolves* further enrich this exploration by providing context and real-life examples of how these scientific principles play out in everyday experiences. These texts have helped shape our current understanding of BPD and continue to influence both clinical practice and personal journeys toward healing.

As we move forward, the insights gained from this scientific inquiry will serve as the backbone for subsequent chapters. With a clearer understanding of the biological and psychological foundations of BPD, we are better equipped to explore how these insights translate into therapeutic interventions and practical strategies for managing the disorder. The integration of science and personal narrative is not merely an academic exercise—it is a pathway to empowerment, offering hope that through understanding, one can learn to navigate even the most turbulent emotional landscapes.

Ultimately, the exploration of the science behind BPD reinforces a fundamental truth: while the disorder may have its roots in our biology and early experiences, it does not define our future. With the right combination of therapeutic techniques, self-compassion, and scientific insight, women with BPD can chart a course toward resilience and recovery. The journey is challenging, but each step taken in understanding the disorder is a step toward reclaiming one's life.

In the chapters that follow, we will build on this foundation by examining the role of trauma and emotional dysregulation, the impact of therapeutic interventions, and the importance of building robust support systems. By continuing to bridge the gap between the scientific and the personal, this book aims to empower readers with the knowledge and strategies needed to live a balanced and fulfilling life despite the challenges of BPD.

Through the detailed examination of the neurological and psychological aspects of BPD presented in this chapter, we have established a framework that not only explains the symptoms but also guides us toward effective treatment. As research continues to evolve, so too does our capacity to address the intricate needs of those with BPD—reminding us that every scientific discovery is a stepping stone toward healing and hope.

4

The Role of Trauma and Early Life Experiences

Trauma is often the hidden architect behind the emotional turbulence seen in Borderline Personality Disorder (BPD). In this chapter, we explore how early life experiences—particularly traumatic ones—can lay the groundwork for the development of BPD. We examine the impact of trauma on emotional regulation, attachment, and self-identity, drawing on both clinical research and personal narratives. Along the way, we reference influential texts that have shaped our understanding of trauma, such as The Body Keeps the Score by Bessel van der Kolk, Trauma and Recovery by Judith Herman, and I Hate You, Don't Leave Me by Jerold J. Kreisman and Hal Straus. These works, among others, provide a framework for understanding how adverse early experiences can manifest as lifelong struggles with instability and relational difficulties.

Understanding Trauma: A Fundamental Concept

Trauma is not a singular experience; it encompasses a wide range of events—from physical or sexual abuse to neglect, emotional invalidation, and even the loss of a loved one. When these events occur during critical periods of development, they can profoundly affect brain development, emotional regulation, and the formation of identity. The idea that "the body keeps the score" is central here, as van der Kolk explains in his seminal work. Our bodies and minds record and store these experiences, sometimes long before we can consciously process them, setting the stage for later psychological difficulties.

For many women with BPD, trauma is not an isolated event but a chronic state of emotional turmoil that began in childhood. Early attachment experiences, particularly those involving caregivers who were unable to provide consistent support, can create an internal working model of relationships that is fraught with anxiety and fear of abandonment. Judith Herman, in *Trauma and Recovery*, describes how repeated exposure to traumatic events can erode one's sense of safety and self-worth. These experiences are pivotal, as they lay the foundation for the unstable interpersonal relationships and fluctuating self-identity that are hallmarks of BPD.

The Impact of Childhood Trauma on Emotional Regulation

One of the most striking features of BPD is the difficulty in managing intense emotions. Childhood trauma plays a significant role in the development of this emotional dysregulation. When children experience neglect or abuse, their developing brains often do not learn effective ways to process and cope with strong emotions. Instead, these children may develop a hypersensitive stress response system, which persists into adulthood.

Research has shown that early trauma can lead to changes in brain regions involved in emotion regulation, such as the amygdala and the prefrontal cortex. These neurological changes make it difficult for individuals to manage the flood of emotions that can be triggered by even minor stressors later in life. This connection between early trauma and emotional reactivity is supported by clinical studies and is a recurring theme in both scientific literature and personal accounts from women living with BPD.

For example, many women describe feeling overwhelmed by emotions that seem disproportionate to the events that trigger them. They often report that their bodies react with anxiety, anger, or despair without a clear rational cause—responses that are, in many ways, echoes of earlier traumatic experiences. This phenomenon underscores the importance of trauma-informed care in treating BPD, as understanding the roots of emotional dysregulation is essential for developing effective therapeutic strategies.

Attachment Disruptions and Their Long-Term Effects

Attachment theory offers a robust framework for understanding how early relationships shape our emotional lives. Secure attachment in childhood provides a stable base from which a child can explore the world and develop self-confidence. However, when a child's early relationships are characterized by inconsistency, neglect, or abuse, the resulting insecure attachment can lead to profound long-term effects.

Women with BPD often report chaotic early relationships where caregivers were either emotionally unavailable or erratic in their responses. This inconsistency leads to an internal conflict: a deep-seated need for closeness and validation coupled with a paralyzing fear of abandonment. In *I Hate You, Don't Leave Me*, Kreisman and Straus vividly illustrate how these early relational disruptions can result in a pattern of idealizing and then devaluing relationships—a cycle that is both painful and self-perpetuating.

The impact of disrupted attachment is multifaceted. Not only does it contribute to difficulties in forming stable relationships, but it also affects the development of self-identity. When caregivers fail to provide a consistent mirror of the child's worth, the child may struggle to form a coherent sense of self. This fragmented self-image often persists into adulthood, manifesting as identity disturbances and an inability to regulate emotions effectively. Such experiences help explain why many women with BPD feel as though they are constantly in a state of flux, never quite sure of who they are or what they deserve.

The Cycle of Trauma and Its Perpetuation in Relationships

Trauma does not occur in isolation; it can set off a chain reaction that affects every aspect of an individual's life, particularly interpersonal relationships. Women with BPD often find themselves caught in a cycle where early trauma shapes their perceptions of relationships, leading to behaviors that inadvertently recreate those early dynamics. This cycle is characterized by intense, unstable relationships marked by extreme shifts in perception—from deep love and admiration to intense anger and rejection.

In *Stop Walking on Eggshells*, Mason and Kreger explore how the fear of abandonment and the instability of early attachments can lead to a pattern of push-pull dynamics in relationships. This oscillation between idealization and devaluation not only causes significant distress for the individual with BPD but also places a heavy emotional burden on their loved ones. The cycle of trauma is thus perpetuated, as each unstable relationship reinforces the individual's internalized belief that relationships are inherently unpredictable and unsafe.

Breaking this cycle is one of the primary goals of trauma-informed therapy. By recognizing and addressing the lingering effects of early trauma, individuals with BPD can begin to develop healthier, more stable ways of relating to others. Therapeutic approaches such as Dialectical Behavior Therapy (DBT) and trauma-focused cognitive-behavioral therapy (TF-CBT) have shown promise in helping women untangle the complex web of past traumas and current relational patterns. These therapies provide not only strategies for managing emotional dysregulation but also tools for building more secure, validating relationships.

The Intersection of Trauma, Identity, and Self-Perception

Trauma's impact extends beyond emotional regulation and interpersonal relationships—it also profoundly influences one's sense of self. A significant aspect of BPD is the struggle with identity, where individuals experience a fragmented or unstable sense of who they are. Early traumatic experiences can shatter a child's developing identity, leaving behind a legacy of self-doubt and internal conflict.

In many cases, women with BPD describe a persistent feeling of emptiness or a lack of core identity—a void that seems impossible to fill. This phenomenon is often rooted in early experiences of invalidation, where the child's feelings and needs were consistently dismissed or minimized by caregivers. Over time, the absence of external validation can lead to an internalized belief that one's true self is unworthy or unlovable.

Clarissa Pinkola Estés' *Women Who Run with the Wolves* delves into the idea of reclaiming the wild, authentic self that has been suppressed by societal expectations. While not solely focused on BPD, Estés' work resonates with many women who have experienced trauma. Her narrative invites readers to reconnect with the parts of themselves that have been lost or overshadowed by pain. For many women with BPD, the journey toward healing involves a process of rediscovering and reclaiming their true identity—a process that is as much about self-compassion as it is about therapeutic intervention.

Therapeutic Approaches to Healing Trauma

Given the deep-rooted nature of trauma in the development of BPD, addressing these early experiences is crucial for recovery. Modern therapeutic approaches increasingly emphasize the need for trauma-informed care—a perspective that prioritizes understanding the role of past trauma in current symptoms and behaviors.

Trauma-Focused Therapies

Trauma-focused therapies, such as Eye Movement Desensitization and Reprocessing (EMDR) and Trauma-Focused Cognitive Behavioral Therapy (TF-CBT), aim to help individuals process and integrate traumatic memories in a way that reduces their emotional charge. EMDR, for instance, has been shown to be effective in alleviating the distress associated with traumatic memories by helping the brain reprocess these events in a more adaptive manner. These approaches are particularly beneficial for women with BPD, as they address both the cognitive and emotional dimensions of trauma.

In *The Body Keeps the Score*, van der Kolk outlines how trauma-focused therapies can help rewire the brain's response to stress and emotional triggers. By engaging with traumatic memories in a safe and controlled environment, individuals can begin to dismantle the patterns of emotional reactivity that have defined their lives. This process is not quick or easy, but it offers a pathway toward healing that acknowledges the deep-seated impact of trauma.

Integrating Mindfulness and Self-Compassion

Mindfulness-based therapies, which are a cornerstone of Dialectical Behavior Therapy (DBT), also play a critical role in healing trauma. Mindfulness practices encourage individuals to become aware of their thoughts and emotions without judgment, creating a space for reflection and self-compassion. By learning to observe their internal experiences without becoming overwhelmed, women with BPD can begin to break free from the automatic, trauma-induced reactions that have long governed their lives.

Books like *The Buddha and the Borderline* highlight the transformative power of mindfulness in the context of BPD. These texts show how mindfulness and self-compassion can help individuals develop a kinder, more forgiving relationship with themselves. Over time, these practices can erode the rigid, negative self-perceptions that are often the legacy of early trauma.

Building a Supportive Therapeutic Relationship

A crucial aspect of healing from trauma is the development of a supportive therapeutic relationship. For many women with BPD, past experiences of betrayal and abandonment have left deep scars that make trusting others challenging. However, the therapeutic alliance—built on empathy, consistency, and validation—can be a powerful antidote to the isolation and mistrust fostered by early trauma.

In *I Hate You, Don't Leave Me*, Kreisman and Straus discuss the importance of having a reliable support system. This is echoed in therapeutic settings where clinicians work collaboratively with patients, ensuring that they feel seen, heard, and valued. Establishing such a bond is essential not only for processing trauma but also for fostering a sense of security that can generalize to other relationships outside of therapy.

Personal Narratives: Voices from the Journey

No discussion of trauma and BPD would be complete without acknowledging the personal narratives of those who have lived through these experiences. Many women with BPD share common threads in their stories—a profound sense of early loss, chronic feelings of abandonment, and a lifelong struggle to define their own worth. These stories serve as a powerful reminder that while the scars of trauma are deep, healing is possible.

One composite narrative we encounter is that of Maya, who describes her childhood as a constant state of uncertainty. Abandoned emotionally by caregivers who were ill-equipped to meet her needs, Maya grew up feeling both desperate for connection and terrified of intimacy. Her adult relationships mirrored this push-pull dynamic, oscillating between intense longing and acute fear of being hurt. Through therapy, Maya gradually began to understand how her early trauma had shaped her behavior. With the support of a compassionate therapist and a commitment to mindfulness practices, she embarked on a journey toward reclaiming her identity and building healthier relationships.

Maya's story, like those documented in many case studies and personal accounts, reinforces the idea that the path to healing from trauma is neither linear nor uniform. Every journey is unique, and while the scars of the past may never completely fade, they can become less defining with the right interventions and supports.

Moving Toward Integration and Healing

The process of healing from trauma is as multifaceted as the trauma itself. For women with BPD, recovery often means learning to integrate fragmented parts of the self, acknowledging the pain of the past without allowing it to dictate the future. This integration is not merely about suppressing traumatic memories but about weaving them into a broader narrative of resilience and growth.

The journey toward healing involves multiple layers: acknowledging the trauma, understanding its impact on one's emotional and relational life, and gradually learning to create new, healthier patterns of behavior. It is a process that requires patience, courage, and above all, self-compassion. Books like *Women Who Run with the Wolves* offer a poetic yet profound reminder that the process of reclaiming one's true self is both a challenge and a celebration of life's inherent strength.

Conclusion

In this chapter, we have explored how trauma and early life experiences contribute to the development and persistence of BPD. From the neurological changes that underlie emotional dysregulation to the deep-seated attachment issues that shape relational patterns, the evidence is clear: early trauma casts a long shadow over an individual's emotional life. Yet, within this shadow lies the potential for transformation—a chance to understand, heal, and ultimately reclaim one's life.

The insights drawn from seminal texts such as *The Body Keeps the Score*, *Trauma and Recovery*, and *I Hate You, Don't Leave Me* provide both a scientific and humanistic perspective on trauma. They remind us that while the legacy of early pain is profound, it is not insurmountable. With the right therapeutic approaches— be it trauma-focused therapy, mindfulness, or the nurturing of a supportive therapeutic alliance—women with BPD can begin to heal the wounds of the past and forge a path toward a more balanced and resilient future.

As we move forward in this book, the themes of trauma, recovery, and resilience will continue to surface. The next chapters will build upon this foundation by exploring how therapeutic interventions can further empower women to manage BPD, establish healthier relationships, and reclaim their identities. The journey through trauma is challenging, but it is also a journey toward rediscovering the inherent strength and capacity for transformation that lies within every individual.

Ultimately, understanding the role of trauma in BPD is not just about identifying past wounds—it is about recognizing the possibilities for healing that emerge when we confront those wounds with compassion, insight, and a commitment to change. In doing so, we honor both the pain of the past and the promise of a more hopeful future.

By integrating clinical research, psychological theory, and the lived experiences of women who have navigated the complexities of early trauma, this chapter provides a comprehensive look at how trauma shapes the landscape of BPD. The works of van der Kolk, Herman, Kreisman, and others enrich our understanding, offering both a diagnosis of the problem and a glimpse at the solutions that lie ahead. As we continue to explore the multifaceted world of BPD in subsequent chapters, the lessons of trauma and recovery will remain a central, guiding force in the journey toward healing and self-discovery.

Trauma is often the hidden architect behind the emotional turbulence seen in Borderline Personality Disorder (BPD). In this chapter, we explore how early life experiences—particularly traumatic ones—can lay the groundwork for the development of BPD. We examine the impact of trauma on emotional regulation, attachment, and self-identity, drawing on both clinical research and personal narratives. Along the way, we reference influential texts that have shaped our understanding of trauma, such as *The Body Keeps the Score* by Bessel van der Kolk, *Trauma and Recovery* by Judith Herman, and *I Hate You, Don't Leave Me* by Jerold J. Kreisman and Hal Straus. These works, among others, provide a framework for understanding how adverse early experiences can manifest as lifelong struggles with instability and relational difficulties.

Understanding Trauma: A Fundamental Concept

Trauma is not a singular experience; it encompasses a wide range of events—from physical or sexual abuse to neglect, emotional invalidation, and even the loss of a loved one. When these events occur during critical periods of development, they can profoundly affect brain development, emotional regulation, and the formation of identity. The idea that "the body keeps the score" is central here, as van der Kolk explains in his seminal work. Our bodies and minds record and store these experiences, sometimes long before we can consciously process them, setting the stage for later psychological difficulties.

For many women with BPD, trauma is not an isolated event but a chronic state of emotional turmoil that began in childhood.

Early attachment experiences, particularly those involving caregivers who were unable to provide consistent support, can create an internal working model of relationships that is fraught with anxiety and fear of abandonment. Judith Herman, in *Trauma and Recovery*, describes how repeated exposure to traumatic events can erode one's sense of safety and self-worth. These experiences are pivotal, as they lay the foundation for the unstable interpersonal relationships and fluctuating self-identity that are hallmarks of BPD.

The Impact of Childhood Trauma on Emotional Regulation

One of the most striking features of BPD is the difficulty in managing intense emotions. Childhood trauma plays a significant role in the development of this emotional dysregulation. When children experience neglect or abuse, their developing brains often do not learn effective ways to process and cope with strong emotions. Instead, these children may develop a hypersensitive stress response system, which persists into adulthood.

Research has shown that early trauma can lead to changes in brain regions involved in emotion regulation, such as the amygdala and the prefrontal cortex. These neurological changes make it difficult for individuals to manage the flood of emotions that can be triggered by even minor stressors later in life. This connection between early trauma and emotional reactivity is supported by clinical studies and is a recurring theme in both scientific literature and personal accounts from women living with BPD.

For example, many women describe feeling overwhelmed by emotions that seem disproportionate to the events that trigger them. They often report that their bodies react with anxiety, anger, or despair without a clear rational cause—responses that are, in many ways, echoes of earlier traumatic experiences. This phenomenon underscores the importance of trauma-informed care in treating BPD, as understanding the roots of emotional dysregulation is essential for developing effective therapeutic strategies.

Attachment Disruptions and Their Long-Term Effects

Attachment theory offers a robust framework for understanding how early relationships shape our emotional lives. Secure attachment in childhood provides a stable base from which a child can explore the world and develop self-confidence. However, when a child's early relationships are characterized by inconsistency, neglect, or abuse, the resulting insecure attachment can lead to profound long-term effects.

Women with BPD often report chaotic early relationships where caregivers were either emotionally unavailable or erratic in their responses. This inconsistency leads to an internal conflict: a deep-seated need for closeness and validation coupled with a paralyzing fear of abandonment. In *I Hate You, Don't Leave Me*, Kreisman and Straus vividly illustrate how these early relational disruptions can result in a pattern of idealizing and then devaluing relationships—a cycle that is both painful and self-perpetuating.

The impact of disrupted attachment is multifaceted. Not only does it contribute to difficulties in forming stable relationships, but it also affects the development of self-identity. When caregivers fail to provide a consistent mirror of the child's worth, the child may struggle to form a coherent sense of self. This fragmented self-image often persists into adulthood, manifesting as identity disturbances and an inability to regulate emotions effectively. Such experiences help explain why many women with BPD feel as though they are constantly in a state of flux, never quite sure of who they are or what they deserve.

The Cycle of Trauma and Its Perpetuation in Relationships

Trauma does not occur in isolation; it can set off a chain reaction that affects every aspect of an individual's life, particularly interpersonal relationships. Women with BPD often find themselves caught in a cycle where early trauma shapes their perceptions of relationships, leading to behaviors that inadvertently recreate those early dynamics. This cycle is characterized by intense, unstable relationships marked by extreme shifts in perception—from deep love and admiration to intense anger and rejection.

In *Stop Walking on Eggshells*, Mason and Kreger explore how the fear of abandonment and the instability of early attachments can lead to a pattern of push-pull dynamics in relationships. This oscillation between idealization and devaluation not only causes significant distress for the individual with BPD but also places a heavy emotional burden on their loved ones. The cycle of trauma is thus perpetuated, as each unstable relationship reinforces the individual's internalized belief that relationships are inherently unpredictable and unsafe.

Breaking this cycle is one of the primary goals of trauma-informed therapy. By recognizing and addressing the lingering effects of early trauma, individuals with BPD can begin to develop healthier, more stable ways of relating to others. Therapeutic approaches such as Dialectical Behavior Therapy (DBT) and trauma-focused cognitive-behavioral therapy (TF-CBT) have shown promise in helping women untangle the complex web of past traumas and current relational patterns. These therapies provide not only strategies for managing emotional dysregulation but also tools for building more secure, validating relationships.

The Intersection of Trauma, Identity, and Self-Perception

Trauma's impact extends beyond emotional regulation and interpersonal relationships—it also profoundly influences one's sense of self. A significant aspect of BPD is the struggle with identity, where individuals experience a fragmented or unstable sense of who they are. Early traumatic experiences can shatter a child's developing identity, leaving behind a legacy of self-doubt and internal conflict.

In many cases, women with BPD describe a persistent feeling of emptiness or a lack of core identity—a void that seems impossible to fill. This phenomenon is often rooted in early experiences of invalidation, where the child's feelings and needs were consistently dismissed or minimized by caregivers. Over time, the absence of external validation can lead to an internalized belief that one's true self is unworthy or unlovable.

Clarissa Pinkola Estés' *Women Who Run with the Wolves* delves into the idea of reclaiming the wild, authentic self that has been suppressed by societal expectations. While not solely focused on BPD, Estés' work resonates with many women who have experienced trauma. Her narrative invites readers to reconnect with the parts of themselves that have been lost or overshadowed by pain. For many women with BPD, the journey toward healing involves a process of rediscovering and reclaiming their true identity—a process that is as much about self-compassion as it is about therapeutic intervention.

Therapeutic Approaches to Healing Trauma

Given the deep-rooted nature of trauma in the development of BPD, addressing these early experiences is crucial for recovery. Modern therapeutic approaches increasingly emphasize the need for trauma-informed care—a perspective that prioritizes understanding the role of past trauma in current symptoms and behaviors.

Trauma-Focused Therapies

Trauma-focused therapies, such as Eye Movement Desensitization and Reprocessing (EMDR) and Trauma-Focused Cognitive Behavioral Therapy (TF-CBT), aim to help individuals process and integrate traumatic memories in a way that reduces their emotional charge. EMDR, for instance, has been shown to be effective in alleviating the distress associated with traumatic memories by helping the brain reprocess these events in a more adaptive manner. These approaches are particularly beneficial for women with BPD, as they address both the cognitive and emotional dimensions of trauma.

In *The Body Keeps the Score*, van der Kolk outlines how trauma-focused therapies can help rewire the brain's response to stress and emotional triggers. By engaging with traumatic memories in a safe and controlled environment, individuals can begin to dismantle the patterns of emotional reactivity that have defined their lives. This process is not quick or easy, but it offers a pathway toward healing that acknowledges the deep-seated impact of trauma.

Integrating Mindfulness and Self-Compassion

Mindfulness-based therapies, which are a cornerstone of Dialectical Behavior Therapy (DBT), also play a critical role in healing trauma. Mindfulness practices encourage individuals to become aware of their thoughts and emotions without judgment, creating a space for reflection and self-compassion. By learning to observe their internal experiences without becoming overwhelmed, women with BPD can begin to break free from the automatic, trauma-induced reactions that have long governed their lives.

Books like *The Buddha and the Borderline* highlight the transformative power of mindfulness in the context of BPD. These texts show how mindfulness and self-compassion can help individuals develop a kinder, more forgiving relationship with themselves. Over time, these practices can erode the rigid, negative self-perceptions that are often the legacy of early trauma.

Building a Supportive Therapeutic Relationship

A crucial aspect of healing from trauma is the development of a supportive therapeutic relationship. For many women with BPD, past experiences of betrayal and abandonment have left deep scars that make trusting others challenging. However, the therapeutic alliance—built on empathy, consistency, and validation—can be a powerful antidote to the isolation and mistrust fostered by early trauma.

In *I Hate You, Don't Leave Me*, Kreisman and Straus discuss the importance of having a reliable support system. This is echoed in therapeutic settings where clinicians work collaboratively with patients, ensuring that they feel seen, heard, and valued. Establishing such a bond is essential not only for processing trauma but also for fostering a sense of security that can generalize to other relationships outside of therapy.

Personal Narratives: Voices from the Journey

No discussion of trauma and BPD would be complete without acknowledging the personal narratives of those who have lived through these experiences. Many women with BPD share common threads in their stories—a profound sense of early loss, chronic feelings of abandonment, and a lifelong struggle to define their own worth. These stories serve as a powerful reminder that while the scars of trauma are deep, healing is possible.

One composite narrative we encounter is that of Maya, who describes her childhood as a constant state of uncertainty. Abandoned emotionally by caregivers who were ill-equipped to meet her needs, Maya grew up feeling both desperate for connection and terrified of intimacy. Her adult relationships mirrored this push-pull dynamic, oscillating between intense longing and acute fear of being hurt. Through therapy, Maya gradually began to understand how her early trauma had shaped her behavior. With the support of a compassionate therapist and a commitment to mindfulness practices, she embarked on a journey toward reclaiming her identity and building healthier relationships.

Maya's story, like those documented in many case studies and personal accounts, reinforces the idea that the path to healing from trauma is neither linear nor uniform. Every journey is unique, and while the scars of the past may never completely fade, they can become less defining with the right interventions and supports.

Moving Toward Integration and Healing

The process of healing from trauma is as multifaceted as the trauma itself. For women with BPD, recovery often means learning to integrate fragmented parts of the self, acknowledging the pain of the past without allowing it to dictate the future. This integration is not merely about suppressing traumatic memories but about weaving them into a broader narrative of resilience and growth.

The journey toward healing involves multiple layers: acknowledging the trauma, understanding its impact on one's emotional and relational life, and gradually learning to create new, healthier patterns of behavior. It is a process that requires patience, courage, and above all, self-compassion. Books like *Women Who Run with the Wolves* offer a poetic yet profound reminder that the process of reclaiming one's true self is both a challenge and a celebration of life's inherent strength.

Conclusion

In this chapter, we have explored how trauma and early life experiences contribute to the development and persistence of BPD. From the neurological changes that underlie emotional dysregulation to the deep-seated attachment issues that shape relational patterns, the evidence is clear: early trauma casts a long shadow over an individual's emotional life. Yet, within this shadow lies the potential for transformation—a chance to understand, heal, and ultimately reclaim one's life.

The insights drawn from seminal texts such as *The Body Keeps the Score*, *Trauma and Recovery*, and *I Hate You, Don't Leave Me* provide both a scientific and humanistic perspective on trauma. They remind us that while the legacy of early pain is profound, it is not insurmountable. With the right therapeutic approaches— be it trauma-focused therapy, mindfulness, or the nurturing of a supportive therapeutic alliance—women with BPD can begin to heal the wounds of the past and forge a path toward a more balanced and resilient future.

As we move forward in this book, the themes of trauma, recovery, and resilience will continue to surface. The next chapters will build upon this foundation by exploring how therapeutic interventions can further empower women to manage BPD, establish healthier relationships, and reclaim their identities. The journey through trauma is challenging, but it is also a journey toward rediscovering the inherent strength and capacity for transformation that lies within every individual.

Ultimately, understanding the role of trauma in BPD is not just about identifying past wounds—it is about recognizing the possibilities for healing that emerge when we confront those wounds with compassion, insight, and a commitment to change. In doing so, we honor both the pain of the past and the promise of a more hopeful future.

By integrating clinical research, psychological theory, and the lived experiences of women who have navigated the complexities of early trauma, this chapter provides a comprehensive look at how trauma shapes the landscape of BPD. The works of van der Kolk, Herman, Kreisman, and others enrich our understanding, offering both a diagnosis of the problem and a glimpse at the solutions that lie ahead. As we continue to explore the multifaceted world of BPD in subsequent chapters, the lessons of trauma and recovery will remain a central, guiding force in the journey toward healing and self-discovery.

5

Emotional Dysregulation and Identity Struggles

Borderline Personality Disorder (BPD) is often defined by two interwoven challenges: emotional dysregulation and identity struggles. In this chapter, we explore these interconnected dimensions, delving into how intense emotions can distort one's sense of self and vice versa. We will examine the underlying mechanisms of emotional dysregulation, the role of cognitive distortions, and the often painful journey toward developing a stable identity. Along the way, we draw on seminal works such as I Hate You, Don't Leave Me by Jerold J. Kreisman and Hal Straus, Stop Walking on Eggshells by Paul Mason and Randi Kreger, Women Who Run with the Wolves by Clarissa Pinkola Estés, and The Buddha and the Borderline by Kiera Van Gelder, all of which have provided invaluable insights into these struggles and the paths to healing.

The Nature of Emotional Dysregulation

Understanding the Intensity of Emotions

At the heart of BPD lies an emotional landscape that is both vivid and volatile. Emotional dysregulation refers to the difficulty in managing and responding to intense emotions in a controlled manner. For many women with BPD, feelings can surge rapidly—from profound joy to crushing despair—with little warning. This emotional roller coaster is not simply a matter of "being moody"; rather, it represents a fundamental difference in how the brain processes and reacts to stimuli.

Neuroscientific research suggests that the amygdala—the brain's emotional processing center—can be hyper-responsive in individuals with BPD. This hyperactivity means that even minor events can trigger overwhelming feelings. In contrast, the prefrontal cortex, responsible for executive function and impulse control, may not always adequately moderate these reactions. As a result, emotional responses become amplified and difficult to regulate, leading to impulsive actions and volatile interpersonal dynamics.

Cognitive Distortions and Their Impact

Emotional dysregulation is compounded by cognitive distortions—patterns of thinking that tend to exaggerate negative emotions and experiences. These distortions can include black-and-white thinking, catastrophizing, and an overgeneralization of events. For instance, a small disagreement with a loved one may be interpreted as a sign of impending abandonment or rejection. Such thoughts can intensify feelings of worthlessness or anger, fueling a cycle of emotional turmoil.

I Hate You, Don't Leave Me vividly illustrates how these cognitive distortions manifest in real life, portraying the relentless internal battle where emotions override reason. The book explains that the intensity of these emotions can distort perceptions, making it challenging for individuals to see situations clearly. As these cognitive distortions take hold, they reinforce the emotional dysregulation that is central to BPD, creating a self-perpetuating cycle that is difficult to break without targeted therapeutic intervention.

Therapeutic Strategies for Managing Emotions

Interventions such as Dialectical Behavior Therapy (DBT) have been developed to address emotional dysregulation by teaching skills in mindfulness, distress tolerance, emotion regulation, and interpersonal effectiveness. DBT encourages patients to acknowledge their emotions without judgment and to practice techniques that allow them to observe and manage these feelings more effectively. Kiera Van Gelder's *The Buddha and the Borderline* provides a powerful account of how mindfulness and self-compassion can transform the experience of overwhelming emotions. By learning to ground themselves in the present moment, individuals with BPD can begin to mitigate the intense emotional responses that have long dictated their behavior.

Identity Struggles: The Search for a Coherent Self

The Crisis of Self-Identity

Alongside emotional dysregulation, many women with BPD grapple with a profound crisis of identity. This struggle manifests as a persistent uncertainty about who they are, what they value, and what they want from life. The instability of self-image is not just an abstract concept—it directly influences decisions, relationships, and overall well-being. When identity is fluid or fragmented, it becomes nearly impossible to build a stable life foundation.

The roots of identity struggles often trace back to early developmental experiences. In environments marked by inconsistency, neglect, or invalidation, the process of forming a secure sense of self can be disrupted. When caregivers fail to provide a consistent mirror for the child's emotional experiences, the result is often a fragmented self-concept that persists into adulthood. This notion is well articulated in *Stop Walking on Eggshells*, which discusses how an unstable self-image can lead to erratic behaviors and an ongoing crisis in relationships. The text emphasizes that without a solid sense of identity, even everyday decisions can become sources of anxiety and self-doubt.

The Role of Societal Expectations

For many women, societal expectations further complicate the struggle for identity. Cultural norms often impose rigid roles and standards—demanding a balance between being nurturing and independent, strong and delicate—which can be contradictory and overwhelming. The pressure to conform to these ideals can lead women with BPD to feel as if they are constantly failing to live up to an idealized version of themselves. Clarissa Pinkola Estés, in *Women Who Run with the Wolves*, explores the archetypal narratives that shape women's identities. Estés argues that women are often forced to repress their authentic selves in favor of socially acceptable personas, which can exacerbate feelings of emptiness and disconnection.

This tension between the inner self and external expectations is a key component of the identity struggles experienced by women with BPD. When the self is continually fractured by the need to meet external demands, it becomes increasingly challenging to establish an authentic identity. The constant battle between who one is and who one is expected to be creates an inner conflict that fuels both emotional dysregulation and chronic dissatisfaction.

Reclaiming and Reinventing the Self

Despite these profound challenges, the journey toward re-claiming a stable identity is not only possible—it can also be transformative. Therapeutic interventions often focus on helping individuals explore and embrace all facets of their identity. In DBT, for instance, part of the therapeutic process involves validating the individual's emotional experiences while also challenging the harmful cognitive distortions that hinder the development of a coherent self-image.

Books such as *Women Who Run with the Wolves* offer a metaphorical and practical roadmap for reclaiming one's wild, authentic self. Estés' work encourages women to reconnect with the parts of themselves that have been suppressed or overlooked by societal expectations. This process of self-reclamation is both courageous and necessary, providing a foundation upon which a more resilient and genuine identity can be built. By acknowledging the full spectrum of their emotional experiences—both the light and the dark—women with BPD can begin to construct a self-image that is both nuanced and empowering.

Integrating Past and Present

A critical aspect of overcoming identity struggles in BPD is the integration of past experiences with the present. Many women find that their sense of identity is mired in the trauma of their past—memories of neglect, abuse, or invalidation that have become inextricably linked with their self-concept. The process of healing involves not only addressing these past wounds but also learning to integrate them into a broader narrative of resilience and growth.

Therapeutic approaches such as narrative therapy encourage individuals to view their lives as evolving stories rather than fixed identities. By reframing their past experiences, individuals can shift from a perspective of victimhood to one of agency and strength. *The Buddha and the Borderline* illustrates this transformative process, showing how mindfulness and narrative reframing can help women reinterpret their traumatic histories in a way that fosters healing rather than self-blame. This integration of past and present is essential for developing a coherent and resilient identity that can withstand the emotional storms characteristic of BPD.

Intersections: Emotional Dysregulation and Identity

The Vicious Cycle

Emotional dysregulation and identity struggles are deeply intertwined, each exacerbating the other in a vicious cycle. When intense emotions overwhelm an unstable sense of self, it becomes difficult to form and maintain lasting relationships or to make consistent, value-driven decisions. For example, a sudden surge of anger or despair might lead an individual to act in ways that conflict with their long-term values, reinforcing feelings of guilt and further destabilizing their self-image. Conversely, the persistent uncertainty about one's identity can make emotional experiences feel even more overwhelming, as there is no solid foundation from which to draw stability or perspective.

This cycle is poignantly described in *I Hate You, Don't Leave Me*, where personal narratives reveal how emotional highs and lows are often mirrored by fluctuations in self-perception. The book demonstrates that without intervention, the feedback loop between emotional dysregulation and identity fragmentation can lead to increasingly chaotic and self-destructive patterns of behavior.

Breaking the Cycle Through Therapy

Breaking this destructive cycle requires interventions that address both emotional regulation and identity formation simultaneously. DBT, with its emphasis on mindfulness and validation, offers a dual approach: it helps individuals manage their emotional responses while also encouraging self-reflection and the development of a more stable identity. By learning to observe their emotional reactions without immediate judgment, individuals can begin to understand the triggers and patterns that underlie their behavior. This self-awareness is the first step toward reconstructing a coherent self-image that is resilient in the face of emotional turbulence.

Moreover, group therapy settings provide a supportive environment where individuals can share their experiences and learn from one another. In these groups, participants often discover that they are not alone in their struggles—an insight that can be both comforting and empowering. The shared stories, as seen in *Stop Walking on Eggshells*, highlight that many of the challenges associated with BPD are common, and that healing is possible through mutual support and understanding. The collaborative nature of group therapy reinforces the idea that identity is not a solitary construct but one that is continually shaped and reshaped by interpersonal relationships.

The Road to Self-Discovery

Cultivating Self-Awareness

A significant milestone on the path to healing is the cultivation of self-awareness. Self-awareness allows individuals to recognize and understand their emotional patterns and the underlying beliefs that drive their behaviors. This process often begins with mindfulness practices—techniques that help individuals remain present and observe their thoughts and emotions without immediate reaction. Over time, mindfulness can provide the clarity needed to disentangle complex emotional responses from core aspects of identity.

Kiera Van Gelder's *The Buddha and the Borderline* offers practical insights into how mindfulness practices can foster self-awareness and facilitate the integration of fragmented aspects of the self. By regularly engaging in mindfulness meditation and reflective practices, individuals can begin to chart the fluctuations in their emotional landscape, identify recurring triggers, and develop strategies to counteract negative cognitive distortions.

Embracing Vulnerability and Authenticity

Emotional healing often necessitates embracing vulnerability—a concept that many find counterintuitive in a society that prizes strength and stoicism. For women with BPD, vulnerability is not a weakness but a pathway to authenticity. Accepting vulnerability means acknowledging the full range of one's emotions and experiences, including the painful and the joyous, the light and the dark. This acceptance paves the way for a more integrated and resilient identity.

Clarissa Pinkola Estés, in *Women Who Run with the Wolves*, advocates for the reclamation of the wild, unfiltered self—a self that has often been suppressed by external pressures and internalized criticism. By embracing vulnerability, individuals can dismantle the false personas that have been constructed to hide their true selves. This process of stripping away pretense is challenging, yet it is a vital step in forging an identity that is both authentic and robust.

Rebuilding a Coherent Self

The journey to rebuilding a coherent self is gradual and non-linear. It involves piecing together the disparate fragments of one's identity, reconciling conflicting aspects of the self, and ultimately constructing a narrative that acknowledges both past pain and future possibilities. Therapeutic techniques such as narrative therapy encourage individuals to reframe their life stories, emphasizing growth, resilience, and self-empowerment over victimhood. By doing so, individuals begin to see themselves not as defined by their disorder but as whole, complex beings with the capacity for change and renewal.

The integration of therapeutic insights from texts like *Stop Walking on Eggshells* and *I Hate You, Don't Leave Me* helps illuminate this process. These works offer not only clinical explanations for the behaviors associated with BPD but also hope and practical strategies for reclaiming one's identity. They serve as reminders that while the journey toward self-discovery is fraught with challenges, it is also replete with opportunities for profound personal growth.

Conclusion

Emotional dysregulation and identity struggles form the core of the lived experience of BPD, creating a dynamic interplay that can be both debilitating and transformative. In this chapter, we have explored how intense, rapidly shifting emotions can destabilize one's sense of self and how, in turn, an unstable identity can magnify emotional pain. Drawing on insights from seminal works such as *I Hate You, Don't Leave Me*, *Stop Walking on Eggshells*, *Women Who Run with the Wolves*, and *The Buddha and the Borderline*, we have examined the scientific, psychological, and cultural dimensions of these struggles.

Through an exploration of the neurological basis for heightened emotional responses, the cognitive distortions that fuel negative self-perception, and the societal pressures that complicate the journey toward authenticity, we have mapped out the terrain of emotional dysregulation and identity in BPD. Therapeutic approaches, particularly those grounded in mindfulness and DBT, offer a way forward—providing tools to break the cycle of emotional turmoil and build a more stable, integrated self.

The path to healing is not straightforward; it involves acknowledging the pain of the past, understanding the triggers of the present, and courageously forging a future where vulnerability is seen as strength. As women with BPD learn to navigate their emotional landscapes, they are invited to embark on a journey of self-discovery—a journey that transforms chaos into clarity and fragmentation into wholeness.

In the chapters that follow, we will continue to build on these themes by exploring further therapeutic interventions and the importance of building supportive relationships. The insights gained here are not merely academic; they are the foundations upon which real lives are rebuilt. Every step toward self-awareness, every moment of embracing vulnerability, and every instance of reclaiming one's authentic identity is a victory—a testament to the resilience and strength that reside at the heart of the human spirit.

Ultimately, understanding and addressing emotional dysregulation and identity struggles in BPD is about more than managing symptoms—it is about reclaiming the narrative of one's life. With the right tools, support, and insight, women can transform the challenges of BPD into stepping stones toward a life defined not by disorder, but by resilience, authenticity, and the promise of renewal.

By weaving together scientific research, clinical insights, and the rich narratives found in influential texts, this chapter has provided a comprehensive exploration of the interplay between emotional dysregulation and identity struggles in BPD. As you reflect on these ideas, remember that while the journey may be fraught with challenges, it is also filled with the potential for profound transformation and healing.

6

Therapeutic Interventions and Treatment Modalities

Borderline Personality Disorder (BPD) is a multifaceted condition that requires equally nuanced treatment approaches. In this chapter, we explore the array of therapeutic interventions and treatment modalities available for managing BPD. We will examine established therapies such as Dialectical Behavior Therapy (DBT) and Cognitive Behavioral Therapy (CBT), as well as emerging and complementary approaches. Drawing on both scientific research and personal narratives, we also reference seminal works like Cognitive-Behavioral Treatment of Borderline Personality Disorder by Marsha Linehan, Stop Walking on Eggshells by Paul Mason and Randi Kreger, and The Buddha and the Borderline by Kiera Van Gelder, among others. These texts provide not only clinical insights but also practical strategies for recovery and transformation.

Understanding the Landscape of Therapeutic Interventions

The Need for an Integrated Approach

BPD is characterized by intense emotional dysregulation, identity disturbances, and tumultuous interpersonal relationships. Given these complex presentations, no single treatment is likely to work for everyone. Instead, a combination of therapies is often necessary to address the diverse needs of those with BPD. An integrated treatment model might include individual psychotherapy, group therapy, and, in some cases, pharmacotherapy. This holistic approach is supported by decades of clinical research and is consistently recommended in texts such as *Cognitive-Behavioral Treatment of Borderline Personality Disorder* by Marsha Linehan, which laid the groundwork for many modern treatment strategies.

The Role of Personalized Treatment

Every individual with BPD presents a unique constellation of symptoms and challenges. For some, emotional dysregulation is the most disruptive; for others, identity disturbances or interpersonal conflicts take center stage. Personalization of treatment is essential, and clinicians often tailor interventions based on a thorough assessment of the patient's history, current functioning, and treatment goals. This personalized approach is echoed in *Stop Walking on Eggshells*, where the authors stress the importance of adapting therapeutic strategies to fit the individual dynamics of relationships and self-perception.

Dialectical Behavior Therapy (DBT)

Foundations and Core Components

Dialectical Behavior Therapy (DBT) was specifically developed to help individuals with BPD manage their emotions and reduce self-destructive behaviors. DBT combines elements of cognitive-behavioral therapy with mindfulness practices, emphasizing the development of skills in four key areas:

- **Mindfulness:** Cultivating awareness of the present moment to better manage emotional responses.
- **Distress Tolerance:** Learning strategies to endure and survive crises without resorting to harmful behaviors.
- **Emotion Regulation:** Developing techniques to understand and modulate intense emotions.
- **Interpersonal Effectiveness:** Building skills for effective communication and healthier relationships.

Marsha Linehan's groundbreaking work, as detailed in *Cognitive-Behavioral Treatment of Borderline Personality Disorder*, has been instrumental in popularizing DBT. This therapy not only addresses symptom reduction but also aims to foster long-term change by enhancing the patient's capacity to build a life worth living.

DBT in Practice

In practice, DBT often involves a combination of individual therapy sessions and group skills training. This dual approach allows individuals to receive personalized attention while also benefiting from the support and shared experiences of others facing similar challenges. The structured nature of DBT, with its emphasis on measurable goals and systematic skill development, provides a clear roadmap for recovery. Case studies and clinical reports frequently highlight how DBT can lead to significant reductions in self-harm, suicidal ideation, and interpersonal conflicts. Kiera Van Gelder's *The Buddha and the Borderline* further illustrates how the integration of mindfulness and self-compassion within DBT can empower individuals to reclaim control over their emotional lives.

Successes and Challenges

Despite its effectiveness, DBT is not a panacea. Success in DBT requires commitment from both the therapist and the patient, as well as a willingness to engage in what can be a demanding therapeutic process. Some patients may initially resist the structured nature of DBT or find certain skills challenging to master. However, the long-term benefits—including increased emotional stability, improved relationships, and a stronger sense of self—often outweigh these difficulties. The successes and challenges of DBT are frequently discussed in therapeutic communities and are well-documented in both clinical literature and personal narratives, reinforcing its status as a cornerstone of BPD treatment.

Cognitive Behavioral Therapy (CBT) and Related Modalities

The Cognitive Model

Cognitive Behavioral Therapy (CBT) is another well-established intervention for BPD, though it is often adapted specifically for the disorder. CBT focuses on identifying and challenging cognitive distortions—patterns of thinking that contribute to emotional distress and maladaptive behaviors. By restructuring these thought patterns, CBT helps patients develop a more balanced perspective, which in turn can reduce emotional volatility and impulsive behaviors.

Works like *I Hate You, Don't Leave Me* highlight how destructive cognitive patterns, such as black-and-white thinking and catastrophizing, can exacerbate BPD symptoms. CBT aims to break this cycle by teaching patients to recognize these distortions and replace them with more rational, constructive thoughts.

Enhanced CBT and Schema Therapy

In recent years, variations of traditional CBT have been developed to better address the complexities of BPD. Schema Therapy, for instance, integrates elements of CBT with emotion-focused and psychodynamic approaches. It focuses on identifying and modifying deeply ingrained patterns or "schemas" that develop in childhood and contribute to the enduring sense of self-doubt and relational instability characteristic of BPD. This therapeutic approach has shown promise in helping patients understand the origins of their emotional difficulties and develop healthier patterns of thinking and behavior.

Group therapy, often used in conjunction with individual CBT or Schema Therapy, provides additional opportunities for patients to learn from each other's experiences. In *Stop Walking on Eggshells*, the authors emphasize that the collective sharing of experiences in a group setting can foster validation and understanding, both critical components in the recovery process.

Pharmacotherapy: Medications as Adjunctive Treatments

The Role of Medication

While psychotherapy is the cornerstone of treatment for BPD, medications can also play a supportive role. Pharmacotherapy is not used to "cure" BPD but rather to alleviate specific symptoms that may be debilitating. Medications such as selective serotonin reuptake inhibitors (SSRIs), mood stabilizers, and atypical antipsychotics may be prescribed to address symptoms like depression, anxiety, and impulsivity.

Limitations and Considerations

It is important to note that pharmacotherapy for BPD has its limitations. There is no single medication approved specifically for BPD, and the effectiveness of these drugs can vary widely among individuals. Medications are typically most beneficial when combined with robust psychotherapeutic interventions. In *The Buddha and the Borderline*, Van Gelder discusses how medications can sometimes provide a necessary buffer during periods of acute distress, allowing patients to engage more effectively in therapy. However, reliance solely on medication without concurrent therapy often leads to limited improvements.

The Future of Pharmacological Research

Ongoing research continues to explore new pharmacological approaches and combinations that might better target the neurobiological underpinnings of BPD. Advances in neuroimaging and genetics hold promise for more personalized medication regimens in the future. As our understanding of the neurochemical imbalances in BPD deepens, we may see more targeted therapies that offer improved outcomes when integrated with established psychotherapeutic techniques.

Complementary and Emerging Therapies

Mindfulness and Meditation Practices

Beyond traditional psychotherapy and medication, complementary therapies have gained traction as valuable components of a comprehensive treatment plan for BPD. Mindfulness and meditation practices, for instance, have been shown to help individuals regulate their emotions and cultivate a greater sense of self-awareness. These practices are central to DBT and are also widely advocated in works like *The Buddha and the Borderline*. Mindfulness helps patients observe their emotional experiences without immediate reaction, thereby reducing impulsivity and fostering a more measured response to stress.

Art and Expressive Therapies

Expressive therapies, including art therapy, music therapy, and writing therapy, offer creative outlets for processing complex emotions that might be difficult to articulate verbally. These modalities can be particularly effective for individuals who have experienced trauma or who struggle to express their inner experiences through traditional talk therapy. By providing a safe space to explore and externalize emotions, expressive therapies can complement more structured interventions. Although research in this area is still emerging, anecdotal evidence and early clinical studies suggest that these therapies can play a significant role in reducing symptoms and improving overall well-being.

Somatic and Body-Centered Therapies

Somatic therapies, which focus on the connection between the body and mind, are increasingly recognized as effective treatments for BPD, particularly for addressing the lingering effects of trauma. Techniques such as yoga, massage therapy, and biofeedback help patients become more attuned to their physical sensations and learn to regulate their emotional responses. In *The Body Keeps the Score*, Bessel van der Kolk illustrates how trauma is stored in the body and how somatic therapies can be instrumental in releasing this stored tension, ultimately contributing to emotional healing.

Emerging Digital Therapies

With the advent of technology, digital therapies and mobile applications have emerged as innovative tools to support mental health. These platforms can offer supplementary support for those undergoing treatment for BPD by providing access to mindfulness exercises, DBT skills training, and peer support networks. Although digital therapies are still relatively new, early studies indicate that they can be effective adjuncts to traditional therapy, particularly for individuals who may have limited access to in-person care.

Integrating Therapies: A Collaborative Approach

The Importance of a Multidisciplinary Team

Effective treatment for BPD often requires a collaborative, multidisciplinary approach. This team may include psychother- apists, psychiatrists, social workers, and even peer support specialists. By working together, these professionals can cre- ate a comprehensive treatment plan that addresses the full spectrum of the individual's needs. In practice, this might involve coordinating therapy sessions, managing medication, and incorporating complementary therapies—all designed to help the patient achieve a stable and fulfilling life.

The Patient as an Active Participant

Central to the success of any treatment modality is the active involvement of the patient. Recovery from BPD is not a passive process; it requires a willingness to engage, experiment, and sometimes even face uncomfortable truths about one's emo- tional patterns and behaviors. Therapeutic works like *Stop Walk- ing on Eggshells* emphasize the importance of empowerment and self-agency in the recovery process. When patients are encouraged to take charge of their healing—by tracking their moods, practicing skills, and sharing their experiences—they are more likely to see lasting improvements.

Overcoming Barriers to Treatment

Barriers to effective treatment can range from societal stigma and financial constraints to personal resistance and fear of vulnerability. Clinicians and support networks must work together to create environments where patients feel safe and supported. This might involve community outreach, education campaigns, or simply fostering a therapeutic alliance that is built on trust and respect. By addressing these barriers, more individuals with BPD can access the help they need and embark on a path toward recovery.

Conclusion: The Path Forward

Therapeutic interventions and treatment modalities for BPD represent a dynamic and evolving field. From the established efficacy of DBT and CBT to the promising potential of complementary and emerging therapies, the options available to individuals with BPD continue to expand. While no single treatment is a magic bullet, the integration of multiple approaches—tailored to the individual's unique needs—offers a robust pathway to recovery.

In this chapter, we have examined the diverse treatment options available for BPD, drawing on influential texts such as *Cognitive-Behavioral Treatment of Borderline Personality Disorder*, *Stop Walking on Eggshells*, and *The Buddha and the Borderline.* These works have provided invaluable insights into the complexities of BPD treatment, emphasizing the need for a compassionate, multifaceted approach that empowers individuals to reclaim their lives.

As we look to the future, continued research and innovation

hold promise for even more personalized and effective interventions. The journey toward recovery is ongoing, marked by both challenges and victories. With the right combination of therapeutic support, self-empowerment, and community connection, individuals with BPD can build lives characterized not by the constraints of their diagnosis but by resilience, authenticity, and hope.

Ultimately, the goal of treatment is not just symptom management—it is the transformation of chaos into stability, fragmentation into wholeness, and despair into the promise of a new beginning. The therapeutic interventions discussed in this chapter represent tools on that journey—a journey that, while arduous, is filled with the possibility of renewal and the rediscovery of one's true self.

By weaving together scientific research, clinical insights, and personal narratives from seminal works, this chapter has aimed to provide a comprehensive overview of the treatment modalities available for BPD. It is our hope that the insights shared here will inspire both patients and practitioners to pursue an integrated, patient-centered approach to recovery— one that honors the complexity of BPD while embracing the possibility of a brighter future.

7

The Journey Through Therapy – Case Studies and Personal Growth

The path through therapy is as varied as the individuals who walk it. In this chapter, we delve into the transformative journey of women with Borderline Personality Disorder (BPD) as they navigate the challenges and triumphs of therapy. Through a series of case studies, personal narratives, and reflective insights, we illustrate how structured treatment, self-awareness, and resilience can pave the way for profound personal growth. Drawing on influential texts such as I Hate You, Don't Leave Me by Jerold J. Kreisman and Hal Straus, Stop Walking on Eggshells by Paul Mason and Randi Kreger, and The Buddha and the Borderline by Kiera Van Gelder, we explore the multifaceted nature of recovery—one that is both deeply personal and rooted in evidence-based therapeutic practices.

Embracing the Therapeutic Process

For many women with BPD, the decision to enter therapy is both a courageous and daunting step. The journey begins with acknowledging the need for help and overcoming the stigma and internalized shame that often accompany a diagnosis. The initial phase of therapy can be marked by resistance and vulnerability, as individuals confront long-held beliefs and painful memories. However, this period of early uncertainty is also fertile ground for the seeds of transformation.

Consider the story of Anna, a composite case study representing numerous women who have embarked on the therapeutic path. Anna entered therapy with a profound sense of isolation and self-doubt. Having been labeled "difficult" by previous clinicians, she was initially skeptical of whether any treatment could truly understand her inner turmoil. Through her early sessions, Anna learned that therapy was not a process of simply "fixing" her but rather a journey toward understanding the origins of her intense emotions and fragmented identity.

In *I Hate You, Don't Leave Me*, Kreisman and Straus document similar narratives where clients initially resist the therapeutic process. Their work emphasizes that accepting help is not a sign of weakness but a necessary step toward reclaiming one's agency. For Anna, as for many others, this realization marked the beginning of a gradual shift—from seeing herself as inherently flawed to understanding that her struggles were a response to a lifetime of unprocessed emotions and unmet needs.

Case Studies: Triumphs and Challenges

Anna's Story: From Isolation to Connection

Anna's journey is illustrative of the transformative potential of Dialectical Behavior Therapy (DBT). Initially overwhelmed by emotional turbulence, she struggled with impulsive behaviors and tumultuous relationships. Through DBT's structured skills training, Anna began to develop tools for mindfulness and emotion regulation. In group therapy sessions, she encountered others with similar experiences, and the shared vulnerability in that setting helped her feel less isolated. Over time, Anna started to see progress—not in the form of dramatic overnight changes but as small, steady shifts in how she managed her emotions and engaged in relationships.

Her therapist guided her through exercises that emphasized self-validation and self-compassion, echoing the principles found in *The Buddha and the Borderline*. This book highlights the power of mindfulness as a bridge between self-judgment and self-acceptance. For Anna, each mindful breath and every new DBT skill acquired was a building block toward a more stable sense of self. Her story is a testament to how incremental progress can lead to significant personal growth, even when the road is fraught with setbacks.

Maria's Journey: Integrating Past Trauma with Present Strength

Another composite case study is that of Maria, who entered therapy burdened by the weight of early trauma and chronic emotional instability. Maria's early life was marked by inconsistent caregiving and periods of severe neglect. These formative experiences left her with a pervasive fear of abandonment and an unstable self-image. In therapy, Maria's treatment plan integrated trauma-focused interventions with DBT and Schema Therapy. Through this multi-pronged approach, Maria was able to address both the traumatic roots of her emotional dysregulation and the maladaptive patterns that had taken hold in her relationships.

Her therapist used narrative techniques to help Maria reframe her past. In sessions reminiscent of the approaches discussed in *Stop Walking on Eggshells*, Maria learned to view her traumatic experiences not solely as sources of pain, but as chapters in her story that contributed to her strength and resilience. Over time, Maria began to reclaim parts of her identity that had been obscured by trauma. Her journey was marked by moments of intense emotional release as well as periods of steady growth, illustrating that the process of healing is both nonlinear and deeply personal.

The Role of Peer Support and Group Dynamics

Group therapy has emerged as a vital component in the journey through BPD treatment. In these settings, women find validation in shared experiences, which helps break down the walls of isolation. Group sessions provide a safe space where participants learn that they are not alone in their struggles—a realization that can be incredibly empowering.

In group sessions documented in various case studies, women describe how sharing their stories with peers led to mutual understanding and collective healing. The dynamic of group therapy reinforces that recovery is not only an individual process but also a communal one. These shared experiences, frequently highlighted in *Stop Walking on Eggshells*, underscore the importance of supportive networks. For many women, hearing others articulate similar struggles validates their feelings and encourages a shift from self-criticism to self-acceptance.

Personal Growth and the Evolution of Self-Identity

Therapy is not merely about symptom management—it is about fostering personal growth and rebuilding a coherent identity. For many women with BPD, the journey involves a profound re-examination of who they are and what they value. This process is often painful, as it requires confronting long-held beliefs and reconfiguring a sense of self that has been fractured by years of internal conflict.

The Emergence of Self-Awareness

A cornerstone of personal growth in therapy is the development of self-awareness. Through various therapeutic techniques, individuals begin to recognize the patterns that govern their emotional responses. Mindfulness exercises, reflective journaling, and guided imagery are some of the tools that help women gain clarity about their internal experiences. As illustrated in *The Buddha and the Borderline*, mindfulness is not just a tool for calming the mind; it is a pathway to deeper self-understanding.

Take the example of Sarah, another composite case study, whose journey through therapy was marked by gradual self-discovery. Initially overwhelmed by the chaos of her emotions, Sarah learned to identify triggers and to observe her thoughts without immediate judgment. This newfound self-awareness allowed her to step back from impulsive reactions and to engage more thoughtfully with her inner experiences. As she became more attuned to her emotional landscape, Sarah discovered that she had the capacity to choose her responses rather than be controlled by them. This evolution in self-awareness was pivotal in transforming her identity from one defined by disorder to one characterized by resilience and self-compassion.

Reconstructing Identity Through Narrative

Another key aspect of personal growth in therapy is the reconstruction of one's life narrative. Many women with BPD struggle with a fragmented sense of self—a phenomenon rooted in the disjointed experiences of trauma and emotional volatility. Narrative therapy offers a powerful framework for reassembling these fragments into a coherent story. In this approach, individuals are encouraged to view their lives as evolving narratives rather than static, unchangeable identities.

Maria's case, for example, involved a deep engagement with narrative techniques. With the guidance of her therapist, she began to see her past not as an unalterable series of failures but as a sequence of experiences that, while painful, had also instilled in her a unique strength. This reframing allowed Maria to integrate her past trauma into a broader, more empowering life story. The process of reconstructing one's narrative is beautifully encapsulated in *Women Who Run with the Wolves* by Clarissa Pinkola Estés, which champions the reclamation of the wild, authentic self that lies beneath societal expectations. For Maria and many others, redefining their narrative was not about erasing the past but about embracing it as a source of wisdom and resilience.

The Transformative Power of Vulnerability

One of the most profound insights emerging from therapy is the recognition that vulnerability is not a weakness, but a gateway to genuine connection and growth. For many women with BPD, the fear of vulnerability has been a major barrier to forming healthy relationships—both with others and with themselves. Therapy challenges this notion by encouraging clients to embrace vulnerability as a natural and essential part of the human experience.

Anna's journey, for instance, was marked by moments of courageous vulnerability. As she began to share her fears and insecurities with her therapist and peers, she discovered that opening up led to deeper connections and a more authentic sense of self. This process is echoed in *I Hate You, Don't Leave Me*, where personal narratives reveal that the willingness to be vulnerable often leads to unexpected healing and mutual support. The transformative power of vulnerability lies in its ability to break down the barriers of isolation and to foster a sense of shared humanity.

Reflections on Long-Term Recovery

The journey through therapy is ongoing, and recovery from BPD is rarely a linear process. Setbacks are inevitable, and the path to growth is often marked by both leaps forward and steps back. However, each setback offers an opportunity for learning and deeper insight.

Celebrating Small Victories

One of the critical aspects of long-term recovery is the recognition and celebration of small victories. For many women with BPD, progress may seem incremental—each DBT skill mastered, each moment of self-compassion extended, each time a triggering situation is navigated without self-destructive behavior. These small victories accumulate over time, contributing to a more robust and resilient sense of self. In group therapy settings, sharing these victories reinforces the belief that recovery is possible, and that every step forward, however small, is a testament to one's strength.

The Ongoing Process of Healing

As the therapeutic journey unfolds, it becomes clear that healing is not a destination but a continuous process. The insights gained through therapy often lead to new questions and challenges, prompting a lifelong commitment to self-discovery and growth. Many women find that as they move forward, the tools and strategies they have acquired become part of their daily lives—supporting them through inevitable future challenges.

Therapists emphasize that recovery from BPD is not about

achieving perfection, but about learning to navigate life's com-plexities with greater awareness and resilience. The ongoing process of healing is one of evolution—where old patterns may resurface, but the skills to manage them have grown stronger. This perspective is vital, as it reframes setbacks not as failures but as opportunities to reinforce the progress made.

Conclusion: A Journey of Resilience and Renewal

The journey through therapy, with its myriad challenges and triumphs, is ultimately a journey toward reclaiming one's life. Through case studies like those of Anna, Maria, and Sarah, we have seen how structured therapeutic interventions, combined with personal reflection and vulnerability, can lead to mean-ingful growth. Influential works such as *I Hate You, Don't Leave Me*, *Stop Walking on Eggshells*, *The Buddha and the Borderline*, and *Women Who Run with the Wolves* have provided invaluable insights along this journey, offering both practical guidance and a profound understanding of the human experience.

As women with BPD navigate the intricate pathways of ther-apy, they learn not only to manage their symptoms but to build identities that reflect resilience, authenticity, and hope. The transformative power of therapy lies in its ability to illuminate the way forward—even in the midst of intense emotional storms—and to empower individuals to reclaim the narrative of their lives.

In embracing the journey through therapy, each step—no matter how small—is a testament to the indomitable human spirit. The process of healing, though fraught with challenges, ultimately leads to the discovery of a deeper, more compassion-ate self—a self that is capable of both surviving and thriving.

The stories of those who have walked this path remind us that even in the face of profound adversity, there is always the possibility of renewal and growth.

As we look toward the future, the insights gained from these personal journeys serve as a beacon for those still struggling in the shadows of BPD. They remind us that while the road may be long and winding, it is also filled with opportunities for connection, healing, and transformation. Each shared story, every small victory, and the collective wisdom of therapeutic practice all point toward one clear truth: recovery is not only possible—it is within reach.

By weaving together case studies, reflective insights, and the wisdom gleaned from seminal works, this chapter has offered an in-depth exploration of the therapeutic journey in BPD. The stories of personal growth and transformation illustrate that while the journey through therapy is complex and challenging, it is also a path toward lasting healing and self-discovery. With the right support, tools, and unwavering commitment, women with BPD can transform their lives, turning pain into power and chaos into a renewed sense of self.

In the next chapter, we will shift our focus to the importance of building a support system—exploring how family, friends, and community can play a crucial role in sustaining recovery and fostering long-term well-being. The insights shared here remind us that healing is not a solitary endeavor but a collective journey toward resilience, authenticity, and a brighter future.

8

Building a Support System – Family, Friends, and Community

A robust support system is a cornerstone for healing and resilience, particularly for women managing Borderline Personality Disorder (BPD). While therapy and personal growth strategies are critical, the role of external relationships—be they family, friends, or broader community connections—can significantly influence recovery. In this chapter, we explore the importance of nurturing these supportive relationships, how to overcome common challenges, and practical ways to build a network that not only understands but also actively contributes to your journey of healing. Drawing on insights from seminal works such as *Stop Walking on Eggshells* by Paul Mason and Randi Kreger, *I Hate You, Don't Leave Me* by Jerold J. Kreisman and Hal Straus, and *Women Who Run with the Wolves* by Clarissa Pinkola Estés, we will discuss both the theory and practice behind creating a healthy support system.

The Importance of a Supportive Network

Why Support Matters

For many women with BPD, isolation can be both a symptom and a barrier to recovery. Emotional dysregulation, fear of abandonment, and deep-seated mistrust often leave individuals feeling disconnected and alone. However, research and clinical experience consistently demonstrate that a solid support network can mitigate these challenges by offering validation, understanding, and stability. Social support provides emotional comfort, practical help, and a sense of belonging—elements that are essential for both immediate relief and long-term recovery.

Books like *Stop Walking on Eggshells* emphasize that family members and close friends often struggle to understand BPD, inadvertently reinforcing feelings of alienation. Yet, when educated and engaged properly, these same relationships can become a powerful resource. A supportive network acts as an external anchor during turbulent emotional times, helping individuals to manage stress, reinforce positive behaviors, and celebrate small victories.

The Psychological Impact of Connection

Human beings are inherently social creatures; our emotional well-being is closely linked to the quality of our relationships. When we feel understood and supported, our capacity to cope with stress and emotional pain increases. Conversely, persistent isolation or negative interactions can exacerbate symptoms and lead to deeper feelings of despair. The work of Clarissa

Pinkola Estés in *Women Who Run with the Wolves* reminds us that reconnecting with our authentic selves is not only an internal process—it is also nurtured by the relationships we build and the communities we join. These relationships validate our experiences and encourage us to see our struggles as part of a larger human experience rather than as isolated failures.

Building Support Within the Family

Understanding Family Dynamics

Family relationships can be both a source of strength and a trigger for emotional distress. Many women with BPD report that early family experiences contributed to feelings of instability and invalidation. Dysfunctional family dynamics, such as inconsistent parenting or emotional neglect, may have set the stage for later challenges in trust and self-esteem. However, family members who are willing to learn and adapt can eventually become pillars of support.

Educating family members about BPD is a crucial first step. Resources like *I Hate You, Don't Leave Me* offer families insight into the complex emotional landscape of BPD, shedding light on why certain behaviors occur and how they can help rather than hinder recovery. It is important for family members to understand that BPD is not a moral failing or a choice but a disorder with deep roots in neurobiology and early life experiences.

Strategies for Family Engagement

1. **Education and Communication:**
2. Encourage family members to attend therapy sessions or educational workshops on BPD. Open lines of communication, where everyone feels heard and validated, can gradually rebuild trust.
3. **Setting Boundaries:**
4. Healthy boundaries are essential in any relationship. Family members need guidance on how to support without enabling destructive behaviors. Books like *Stop Walking on Eggshells* suggest that clear, compassionate boundaries can help prevent burnout and resentment on both sides.
5. **Family Therapy:**
6. Family therapy can be particularly effective for addressing longstanding issues and improving dynamics. It offers a safe space where all members can express their feelings and work collaboratively towards healing.

Overcoming Obstacles

Resistance to change within the family is common. Some members may feel overwhelmed or resentful, while others may deny the severity of the disorder. It is important to approach these challenges with empathy and patience. In many cases, gradual change is more sustainable than immediate transformation. The key is to remain consistent in communication and to celebrate small improvements in understanding and behavior.

Cultivating Supportive Friendships

The Role of Friends in Recovery

Friends offer a unique type of support that is both informal and emotionally sustaining. Unlike family, friends are typically chosen based on mutual interests and shared values, which can provide a refreshing contrast to the complexities of familial relationships. For women with BPD, friendships can serve as a mirror for understanding and self-reflection, as well as a source of consistent emotional reinforcement.

According to *I Hate You, Don't Leave Me*, friendships can often become a double-edged sword for those with BPD. The intensity of the disorder sometimes leads to idealization and devaluation of friends, resulting in cyclical conflicts. However, when friendships are nurtured with honesty and mutual respect, they can offer stability and a sense of belonging.

Building and Maintaining Healthy Friendships

1. **Honest Communication:**
2. Open, honest communication is the foundation of any strong friendship. It is vital to express your needs and boundaries clearly, and to encourage your friends to do the same.
3. **Mutual Support:**
4. A friendship is a two-way street. Offer support as much as you seek it. This reciprocity helps build a balanced relationship where both parties feel valued.
5. **Shared Activities:**
6. Engage in activities that promote bonding and mutual en-

joyment. Whether it's a shared hobby or regular meet-ups, these interactions reinforce the connection and provide opportunities for positive experiences.

7. **Managing Conflict:**
8. Conflict is inevitable in any relationship, but it can be managed constructively. Learning conflict resolution skills, as taught in DBT and discussed in *Stop Walking on Eggshells*, can help transform disagreements into opportunities for deeper understanding.

Navigating Challenges

Friendships can be complex, particularly when emotional dysregulation is involved. Misunderstandings may arise quickly, and intense reactions can sometimes push friends away. It is essential to work on self-awareness and mindfulness, so that emotional reactions do not overwhelm rational thought. Over time, learning to regulate these responses can lead to more stable and fulfilling friendships.

Creating Community Connections

The Value of Community

Beyond family and friends, broader community connections play a crucial role in recovery. A community provides a sense of belonging that transcends individual relationships, offering a supportive network that is both diverse and dynamic. Whether it's through support groups, online communities, or local organizations, finding a place where you feel accepted can have profound therapeutic benefits.

Community support can take many forms—from peer-led support groups to community centers that host mental health workshops. Such environments offer a space to share experiences, learn from others, and feel part of something larger than oneself. The narratives in *Women Who Run with the Wolves* remind us that reclaiming our authentic selves often involves reconnecting with the collective wisdom and strength of community.

How to Build Community Connections

1. **Join Support Groups:**
2. Support groups for BPD or mental health challenges provide a structured environment where you can share your experiences and learn from others facing similar struggles. These groups foster empathy, validation, and mutual encouragement.
3. **Engage in Online Communities:**
4. In today's digital age, online forums and social media groups can offer a wealth of support. They provide access to diverse perspectives and immediate feedback, which can be particularly helpful during times of crisis.
5. **Participate in Local Organizations:**
6. Community centers, non-profits, and local mental health organizations often host events and workshops. Participating in these activities not only enhances your support network but also contributes to a sense of purpose and connection.
7. **Volunteer:**
8. Volunteering can be a powerful way to build community bonds while also fostering a sense of self-worth. Con-

tributing to causes that resonate with you creates a positive feedback loop that benefits both your mental health and the community.

Overcoming Social Barriers

For many with BPD, initiating and maintaining community connections can be challenging. Social anxiety, past experiences of rejection, and intense fear of abandonment may hinder efforts to engage with others. Overcoming these barriers often requires stepping out of your comfort zone gradually. Start with small, manageable interactions, and build up to larger social engagements as your confidence grows.

Therapy can also play a supportive role here. Techniques learned in DBT—such as mindfulness and distress tolerance— can help manage the anxiety associated with social interactions. Remember that every small step towards building community is a significant victory in itself.

The Role of Education in Strengthening Support Networks

Educating Yourself and Others

An informed support network is more effective than one that is not. Educating yourself about BPD and sharing that knowledge with family, friends, and community members can demystify the disorder and reduce stigma. Books like *I Hate You, Don't Leave Me* and *Stop Walking on Eggshells* serve as invaluable resources not only for those with BPD but also for their loved ones. When people understand that BPD is a complex condition influenced by biology, trauma, and early relationships, they are better equipped to offer compassionate support.

Communication Tools for Sharing Information

Consider organizing informational sessions or book clubs where you and your support network discuss relevant literature. These gatherings can foster understanding and empathy, making it easier for others to relate to your experiences. Sharing your journey openly not only educates others but also reinforces your own path to healing.

Integrating Support with Professional Treatment

The Synergy of Professional and Personal Support

While building a robust support network outside of therapy is essential, it is most effective when integrated with professional treatment. Therapists can help you navigate difficult relationships, set healthy boundaries, and communicate your needs effectively. In turn, the support you receive from family, friends, and community groups can reinforce the strategies learned in therapy, creating a synergistic effect that enhances overall well-being.

The Role of Peer Support Specialists

Peer support specialists—individuals who have navigated their own mental health challenges—can serve as invaluable guides in building a support system. They offer insights from lived experience and can help bridge the gap between professional treatment and everyday life. Engaging with peer support can also provide a model of recovery, illustrating that healing is not only possible but also sustainable.

Conclusion: Toward a Network of Resilience

In this chapter, we have explored the essential role that a robust support system plays in the recovery from BPD. Family, friends, and community networks are not just external buffers against emotional turmoil—they are active, dynamic contributors to the healing process. By educating those around you, establishing healthy boundaries, and seeking out both in-person and online communities, you can build a network that validates your experiences and encourages your growth.

The journey to building a support system is not without its challenges. Misunderstandings, past traumas, and fears of abandonment can all complicate relationships. However, as the literature in *Stop Walking on Eggshells*, *I Hate You, Don't Leave Me*, and *Women Who Run with the Wolves* suggests, even the most challenging relationships hold the potential for transformation when approached with empathy, patience, and mutual commitment.

By integrating professional guidance with personal efforts to educate and connect, you empower yourself to reclaim not only your emotional stability but also your place in a broader, supportive community. The network you build becomes a testament to your resilience—a tangible reminder that healing, though deeply personal, is also a shared human endeavor.

As you move forward, remember that every step taken toward building supportive relationships is a victory. Whether it's a heartfelt conversation with a family member, a shared moment of understanding with a friend, or a supportive message in an online community, each connection contributes to the larger mosaic of your recovery. Your support system is not just a safety net; it is a dynamic community that celebrates your progress, supports you through setbacks, and ultimately helps you forge a path toward a more fulfilling life.

By weaving together insights from clinical research, personal narratives, and the wisdom of seminal texts, this chapter offers a comprehensive look at the importance of building and maintaining a supportive network. In the next chapter, we will delve into the specifics of navigating interpersonal relationships and setting boundaries—a natural extension of the support system discussed here. With a strong network behind you, you are better equipped to tackle the challenges of relationships and to continue your journey toward lasting healing and self-discovery.

9

Navigating Relationships and Setting Boundaries

Interpersonal relationships are both the crucible and the cata-lyst for personal transformation—especially for women with Borderline Personality Disorder (BPD). The very traits that can foster deep connections, such as emotional intensity and passion, can also lead to volatile and painful interactions if not managed carefully. In this chapter, we explore strategies for navigating relationships and establishing healthy boundaries that honor both individual needs and the dynamics of shared connections. Drawing on clinical insights, personal narratives, and the wisdom of seminal texts like *I Hate You, Don't Leave Me* by Jerold J. Kreisman and Hal Straus, *Stop Walking on Eggshells* by Paul Mason and Randi Kreger, *Women Who Run with the Wolves* by Clarissa Pinkola Estés, and *The Buddha and the Borderline* by Kiera Van Gelder, we will examine practical techniques for managing interpersonal challenges and fostering more stable, respectful connections.

The Complexity of Relationships in BPD

The Double-Edged Nature of Emotional Intensity

One of the defining features of BPD is the capacity for intense emotional experiences. For many women, this sensitivity can lead to profound empathy, passion, and creativity. However, it can also result in impulsive reactions and unpredictable behaviors, which may strain even the most well-intentioned relationships. As Kreisman and Straus describe in *I Hate You, Don't Leave Me*, the oscillation between idealization and devaluation often disrupts interpersonal bonds. These rapid shifts in perception can leave both the individual with BPD and their loved ones feeling hurt and confused.

The challenge lies in harnessing emotional intensity as a strength while minimizing its potential to cause relational turmoil. A key part of this process involves understanding one's triggers and learning how to respond rather than react. Mindfulness practices, as championed in *The Buddha and the Borderline*, offer a pathway to achieving this balance. By becoming more aware of the emotions as they arise, one can begin to modulate reactions and make choices that reflect one's true intentions rather than impulsive outbursts.

The Impact of Attachment Patterns

Early attachment experiences play a significant role in shaping how individuals perceive and interact in relationships. Insecure attachment, often marked by fear of abandonment or rejection, can lead to a cycle of clinging and withdrawal. *Stop Walking on Eggshells* highlights how these patterns can cause individuals to misinterpret neutral or even positive interactions as threats, perpetuating a cycle of emotional instability. Recognizing these patterns is the first step in breaking free from them.

For example, a person with BPD may interpret a friend's need for personal space as a sign of rejection, leading to frantic attempts to re-establish closeness. Over time, these behaviors can wear down relationships, reinforcing the individual's fears and insecurities. By working through these attachment issues in therapy and through self-reflection, individuals can begin to rebuild trust in themselves and in others.

Setting Healthy Boundaries

The Need for Boundaries

Establishing healthy boundaries is a crucial component of maintaining balanced relationships. Boundaries help define where one person ends and another begins—they are the physical, emotional, and psychological lines that protect individual well-being. Without clear boundaries, relationships can quickly become enmeshed or codependent, exacerbating feelings of overwhelm and loss of identity.

As discussed in *Stop Walking on Eggshells*, clear boundaries are essential not only for those living with BPD but also for their loved ones. They provide a framework that supports mutual respect and reduces the likelihood of misunderstandings. Boundaries enable individuals to communicate their needs and limits effectively, creating a space where both parties can flourish.

Practical Strategies for Setting Boundaries

1. **Self-Reflection and Clarity:**
2. Before setting boundaries with others, it is crucial to understand your own needs. Reflect on past experiences and identify situations where you felt overwhelmed or taken advantage of. Journaling or mindfulness practices can help in clarifying what you need from relationships.
3. **Assertive Communication:**
4. Clearly expressing your boundaries is key. Use "I" statements to convey your needs without placing blame. For example, saying, "I need some time to recharge after social events," is more constructive than, "You're overwhelming me."
5. Books like *The Buddha and the Borderline* offer exercises to build assertiveness, teaching techniques to communicate limits compassionately and confidently.
6. **Consistency:**
7. Once boundaries are established, consistency is vital. It can be challenging, especially when emotions run high, but remaining steadfast reinforces your needs and helps others adjust to your expectations.
8. **Flexibility and Reassessment:**
9. Boundaries are not static. They should be flexible enough to adapt as relationships evolve. Regularly reassess your boundaries and adjust them as needed, ensuring they continue to serve your well-being without becoming overly rigid.

Overcoming Resistance

Setting boundaries can sometimes lead to resistance or push-back, particularly from those who are used to blurred or enmeshed interactions. It is important to recognize that this resistance often stems from their own fears and insecurities rather than a reflection of your worth. In *I Hate You, Don't Leave Me*, the authors note that loved ones may initially perceive healthy boundaries as rejection or criticism. Patience, empathy, and clear communication can help mitigate these challenges.

Remember, it is not your responsibility to change others' behavior—only to express your needs and maintain your well-being. Enlisting the support of a therapist or counselor during these transitions can provide valuable guidance and reassurance.

Navigating Interpersonal Dynamics

Understanding Interpersonal Patterns

The dynamics within relationships can be complex and often mirror internal emotional states. Many individuals with BPD experience a pattern of idealizing a person in moments of emotional safety, only to devalue them when fears of abandonment or rejection arise. This cycle can lead to volatile and unpredictable relationships that leave everyone feeling emotionally exhausted.

A key step in navigating these dynamics is developing self-awareness. Recognizing when you are beginning to idealize or devalue someone enables you to pause and reflect on the underlying emotions at play. Techniques from Dialectical

Behavior Therapy (DBT), such as mindfulness and emotional regulation skills, are particularly useful in interrupting these cycles before they escalate.

Strategies for Improving Communication

1. **Active Listening:**
2. Effective communication is a two-way street. Active listening involves fully concentrating on what the other person is saying, validating their feelings, and responding thoughtfully. This practice not only improves mutual understanding but also fosters a deeper sense of connection.
3. **Expressing Vulnerability:**
4. While vulnerability can be frightening, it is also the pathway to genuine intimacy. Sharing your true feelings—when done thoughtfully—invites others to do the same, creating a richer, more authentic connection. *Women Who Run with the Wolves* encourages embracing vulnerability as a source of strength and authenticity.
5. **Conflict Resolution:**
6. Conflicts are inevitable in any relationship. The key is to handle them constructively. Instead of allowing conflicts to escalate into emotional storms, work towards resolving them through calm dialogue and mutual compromise. Learning conflict resolution skills from resources like *Stop Walking on Eggshells* can provide practical tools for managing disagreements without resorting to extremes.
7. **Seeking Feedback:**
8. Honest feedback from trusted friends or family members can be invaluable. It helps you understand how your behavior impacts others and offers opportunities for growth.

Regularly ask for input in a non-defensive way to ensure that your efforts to improve are aligned with the needs of your relationships.

Cultivating Resilience in Relationships

Self-Care as the Foundation

At the heart of navigating relationships successfully is the commitment to self-care. Prioritizing your own mental and emotional well-being is essential before you can fully engage with others. Self-care practices—such as regular exercise, adequate rest, and hobbies that bring joy—serve as a buffer against the emotional turbulence that can arise in interpersonal interactions.

Self-care is not a luxury; it is a necessity. In *The Buddha and the Borderline*, Kiera Van Gelder emphasizes that self-compassion and regular self-care routines are critical for managing the intense emotions associated with BPD. When you care for yourself, you are better equipped to set boundaries, communicate effectively, and maintain healthy relationships.

The Role of Peer Support and Mentorship

In addition to personal relationships, peer support and mentorship play a crucial role in cultivating resilience. Engaging with others who have faced similar challenges can provide a sense of validation and hope. Peer support groups and online communities offer spaces where individuals can share experiences, exchange strategies, and celebrate successes together.

Mentorship, whether formal or informal, provides guidance

and perspective. Learning from someone who has successfully navigated similar relational challenges can inspire and empower you to adopt new ways of interacting and caring for yourself.

Embracing Change and Growth

Healthy relationships evolve over time. As you work on yourself and implement new strategies, you may find that your relationships transform in unexpected ways. Some connections may deepen, while others may naturally drift apart. Accepting these changes as part of your growth is vital.

The transformative journey described in *Women Who Run with the Wolves* is a powerful reminder that growth often involves shedding old patterns and embracing new ways of being. Not every relationship will survive the process of change, but those that do are likely to be more authentic, supportive, and resilient.

Practical Exercises and Reflections

Journaling for Self-Reflection

Journaling is a simple yet effective tool for processing your experiences in relationships. Regularly writing about your interactions, emotions, and reactions can help identify patterns that may be hindering your growth. Reflect on moments when you felt misunderstood or when conflicts escalated—what were the triggers? How might different responses have changed the outcome? Over time, your journal becomes a roadmap for personal growth, offering insights that can inform your approach to future interactions.

Role-Playing Scenarios

Role-playing with a trusted friend or therapist can be a practical way to rehearse new communication strategies. By simulating challenging situations in a safe environment, you can experiment with expressing boundaries, practicing active listening, and managing conflict. These exercises not only build confidence but also provide immediate feedback that is essential for refining your approach.

Mindfulness and Grounding Techniques

Regular mindfulness practice is invaluable for staying present during emotionally charged interactions. Techniques such as deep breathing, progressive muscle relaxation, or guided imagery can help you remain centered, even when emotions threaten to overwhelm you. The mindfulness exercises described in *The Buddha and the Borderline* are particularly effective in reducing the intensity of emotional reactions and allowing for thoughtful responses rather than impulsive reactions.

Conclusion: Toward Healthier, More Fulfilling Relationships

Navigating relationships and setting boundaries is a journey that demands both introspection and active engagement with the world around you. For women with BPD, this process can be particularly challenging due to the interplay of intense emotions and a fragile sense of self. However, by cultivating self-awareness, communicating openly, and establishing clear boundaries, it is possible to create relationships that are not only supportive but also transformative.

As we have explored throughout this chapter, the wisdom found in *I Hate You, Don't Leave Me*, *Stop Walking on Eggshells*, *Women Who Run with the Wolves*, and *The Buddha and the Borderline* offers valuable guidance for turning relational challenges into opportunities for growth. Embracing vulnerability, practicing self-care, and seeking peer support are not just theoretical concepts—they are practical strategies that can help you build a network of relationships that reinforce your journey toward healing.

Remember that each interaction is a learning opportunity. Even when setbacks occur, they provide insight into what works and what needs further adjustment. Over time, with persistence and compassion for yourself and others, you can forge connections that honor your authentic self while nurturing mutual respect and understanding.

In the next chapter, we will shift our focus to self-care and mindfulness, exploring daily practices and routines that empower you to maintain stability and nurture your emotional well-being. With healthy relationships and firm boundaries as your foundation, these self-care strategies will further support your journey toward a balanced, fulfilling life.

By integrating clinical insights, personal narratives, and practical exercises, this chapter has provided a comprehensive exploration of navigating relationships and setting boundaries for women with BPD. The guidance offered here is designed to help transform challenges into stepping stones for growth— fostering connections that are resilient, authentic, and mutually supportive. Every conversation, every boundary set, and every mindful pause is a testament to your ongoing journey toward healthier, more fulfilling relationships.

10

Self-Care and Mindfulness – Tools for Daily Management

Self-care and mindfulness are not luxuries—they are essential tools for managing the emotional turbulence that characterizes Borderline Personality Disorder (BPD). For many women living with BPD, daily life can feel like navigating a storm of intense emotions, impulsive reactions, and overwhelming self-doubt. In this chapter, we will explore how self-care practices and mindfulness techniques can serve as anchors in the midst of this storm. Drawing on insights from seminal works such as *The Buddha and the Borderline* by Kiera Van Gelder, *Women Who Run with the Wolves* by Clarissa Pinkola Estés, *Stop Walking on Eggshells* by Paul Mason and Randi Kreger, and *I Hate You, Don't Leave Me* by Jerold J. Kreisman and Hal Straus, we will outline practical strategies for establishing daily routines that promote stability, self-compassion, and long-term recovery.

The Importance of Self-Care in Daily Management

Redefining Self-Care

Self-care goes beyond occasional pampering or indulgence—it is about consistently attending to your mental, emotional, and physical well-being. For individuals with BPD, self-care can often be neglected due to the overwhelming focus on managing crises and intense emotions. However, establishing a robust self-care routine can provide a steady foundation upon which all other aspects of recovery are built.

As Kiera Van Gelder explains in *The Buddha and the Borderline*, self-care is a form of radical self-respect. It is an act of reclaiming the right to feel safe, valued, and whole. Whether it's through physical exercise, creative pursuits, or simply taking moments to pause and breathe, self-care practices are vital for restoring balance and nurturing resilience.

The Daily Impact of Self-Care

On a day-to-day basis, self-care can transform how you handle stress and emotional triggers. When you make time for activities that replenish your energy and soothe your mind, you create a buffer against the chaos of intense emotions. This daily commitment can help reduce the frequency and severity of mood swings, impulsive behaviors, and relational conflicts that often accompany BPD.

Women Who Run with the Wolves encourages women to recon-nect with their inner wildness and honor their natural rhythms. This reconnection is not about escaping responsibility but about honoring your intrinsic needs and using them as a guide for healthier living. In essence, self-care becomes a vital practice that grounds you in your true self, making it easier to navigate life's challenges.

Mindfulness: The Art of Being Present

What Is Mindfulness?

Mindfulness is the practice of cultivating a non-judgmental, moment-to-moment awareness of your thoughts, feelings, and bodily sensations. This practice is particularly effective for managing BPD because it allows you to observe your internal experiences without immediately reacting to them. Instead of being swept away by intense emotions, you learn to acknowledge them, understand their origins, and choose a more deliberate response.

As detailed in *The Buddha and the Borderline*, mindfulness transforms your relationship with your emotions. Rather than seeing feelings as overwhelming forces that dictate your actions, mindfulness teaches you to view them as transient experiences that you can observe and let pass. This shift in perspective is empowering—it means that while you may not be able to control every emotion that arises, you can control how you respond to it.

Techniques to Cultivate Mindfulness

There are numerous mindfulness techniques that you can incorporate into your daily life. Here are a few practical exercises:

1. **Mindful Breathing:**
2. Begin by focusing your attention on your breath. Notice the sensation of air entering and leaving your nostrils, or the

rise and fall of your chest. If your mind wanders, gently redirect your focus back to your breathing. This simple exercise can be done anywhere and provides an immediate sense of calm.

3. **Body Scan Meditation:**
4. This practice involves mentally scanning your body from head to toe, noticing any sensations, tension, or discomfort without judgment. A body scan not only promotes relaxation but also helps you reconnect with your physical self—a connection that is often disrupted by emotional dysregulation.
5. **Grounding Techniques:**
6. When emotions feel overwhelming, grounding techniques can bring you back to the present moment. One effective method is the "5-4-3-2-1" exercise: identify 5 things you can see, 4 things you can touch, 3 things you can hear, 2 things you can smell, and 1 thing you can taste. This exercise helps shift your focus from emotional distress to sensory awareness.
7. **Mindful Journaling:**
8. Journaling can be a powerful way to process your thoughts and emotions. Rather than simply recording events, try writing about how you feel in the moment, what sensations you notice in your body, and any thoughts that arise. Over time, mindful journaling can reveal patterns in your emotional responses and help you develop a more nuanced understanding of your inner landscape.

Integrating Self-Care and Mindfulness into a Daily Routine

Creating a Personalized Routine

Developing a daily self-care routine is a personal journey, one that requires reflection on what truly nourishes you. Start by identifying activities that help you feel grounded and rejuvenated. For some, this might be a morning meditation session; for others, it might be a walk in nature or a creative hobby like painting or writing.

Consider structuring your day around small, manageable practices that reinforce mindfulness. For example, you might begin with 10 minutes of mindful breathing, followed by a nutritious breakfast, and then a brief journaling session to set your intentions for the day. Over time, these practices can become deeply ingrained habits that provide a stable foundation for your emotional well-being.

Overcoming Barriers to Self-Care

For many individuals with BPD, self-care can feel like an indulgence rather than a necessity. Emotional distress, overwhelming responsibilities, or the belief that self-care is selfish can all serve as barriers. It's important to reframe self-care as an essential component of recovery—not an optional extra.

Books like *Women Who Run with the Wolves* remind us that honoring our needs is a radical act of self-love. When you prioritize self-care, you are not neglecting others; rather, you are ensuring that you have the strength and clarity to show up fully in your relationships and responsibilities. Overcoming these internal barriers may require the support of a therapist or a trusted friend, but the benefits are profound and far-reaching.

Practical Tips for Maintaining Consistency

Consistency is key to reaping the benefits of self-care and mindfulness. Here are some practical strategies to help you stay on track:

- **Schedule Self-Care Time:**
- Treat self-care as an appointment you cannot miss. Put it on your calendar just like any other important commitment.
- **Start Small:**
- If the idea of a long meditation session or an elaborate self-care ritual feels overwhelming, start with just a few minutes a day. Gradually increase the duration as you become more comfortable with the practice.
- **Use Reminders:**
- Set alarms or notifications on your phone to prompt you to take a mindful pause or practice a self-care activity.
- **Create a Supportive Environment:**
- Surround yourself with reminders of self-care—whether it's a journal, a favorite book, or a calming playlist. Your environment can serve as a constant prompt to nurture yourself.
- **Be Flexible:**
- Understand that some days will be more challenging than others. Allow yourself the flexibility to adjust your routine without guilt. Remember, self-care is about nurturing yourself, not imposing rigid expectations.

The Interplay Between Self-Care, Mindfulness, and Recovery

Building Resilience Through Daily Practice

The consistent practice of self-care and mindfulness not only alleviates daily distress but also builds long-term resilience. Over time, these practices help rewire your brain's response to stress, making it easier to manage intense emotions and reduce impulsivity. As you become more adept at recognizing and managing your emotional triggers, you gradually build a reservoir of inner strength that can sustain you through life's inevitable challenges.

Research suggests that mindfulness-based interventions can lead to measurable changes in brain regions associated with emotion regulation, such as the prefrontal cortex and the amygdala. These changes underpin the improved emotional stability observed in many individuals who engage in regular mindfulness practice. By incorporating these practices into your daily routine, you are actively participating in your own neurobiological healing—a process beautifully echoed in *The Buddha and the Borderline*.

Connecting Self-Care with Broader Recovery Goals

Self-care and mindfulness are integral to a broader recovery strategy that encompasses therapy, relationship-building, and community engagement. When you nurture yourself through these practices, you are better able to engage in other aspects of your recovery. For example, maintaining a consistent self-care routine can enhance your ability to set and maintain healthy boundaries in relationships, as discussed in previous chapters.

Moreover, as you cultivate mindfulness, you may find that you are more present and engaged during therapy sessions, group support meetings, and interpersonal interactions. This heightened awareness can lead to deeper insights and more meaningful connections, reinforcing the idea that self-care is not an isolated practice but a central pillar of holistic healing.

Integrating Insights from Influential Works

Lessons from The Buddha and the Borderline

Kiera Van Gelder's *The Buddha and the Borderline* provides both practical exercises and profound insights into how mindfulness can transform the experience of living with BPD. Van Gelder emphasizes that mindfulness is not about eliminating emotions but rather about learning to sit with them, observe them, and allow them to pass without overwhelming you. Her approach is gentle yet powerful, encouraging readers to approach their inner experiences with curiosity and compassion.

Reflections from Women Who Run with the Wolves

Clarissa Pinkola Estés' *Women Who Run with the Wolves* offers a poetic exploration of the wild, untamed aspects of the feminine spirit. Estés challenges us to reconnect with our authentic selves, often suppressed by societal expectations and internalized criticism. Her work underscores that self-care is not merely about physical or mental health—it is about reclaiming your identity and honoring your deepest truths. This holistic perspective can empower you to build a self-care practice that resonates with who you truly are.

Practical Guidance from Stop Walking on Eggshells and I Hate You, Don't Leave Me

Both *Stop Walking on Eggshells* and *I Hate You, Don't Leave Me* offer detailed insights into managing the challenges of BPD, particularly in the context of interpersonal relationships and emotional regulation. These works highlight the importance of self-care as a foundation for building healthier relationships. By taking care of yourself first, you are better equipped to navigate the complexities of human interaction without being overwhelmed by the emotional currents that often accompany BPD.

Personal Stories and Reflections

Anecdotes of Transformation

Throughout the journey of recovery, many individuals have found that even small acts of self-care can have profound effects on their emotional well-being. Consider the story of Lisa, a woman who, after years of feeling engulfed by her emotions, began incorporating a simple daily practice of mindful breathing and journaling. Over time, Lisa noticed that her reactions to stress became less intense, and she felt more capable of handling interpersonal conflicts. Her gradual transformation is a testament to the power of consistency in self-care.

Similarly, many have shared how regular mindfulness practice has enabled them to catch their spiraling thoughts before they lead to impulsive decisions. These personal narratives, echoed in the pages of *The Buddha and the Borderline*, serve as a beacon of hope for anyone struggling to find stability amidst the chaos of BPD.

Reflections on the Process

Adopting self-care and mindfulness practices is not a one-time event—it is a continuous journey of self-discovery and growth. Some days, the practices may seem to yield immediate relief; on other days, the benefits might be more subtle. What remains constant is the gradual accumulation of small victories: moments of calm amidst a storm, insights gleaned from a reflective journal entry, or simply the ability to pause before reacting impulsively.

Each of these moments contributes to a growing sense of self-efficacy—a belief that you can manage your emotions and shape your own recovery. This evolving self-trust is essential for long-term healing and is nurtured by the daily commitment to self-care and mindfulness.

Conclusion: A Foundation for Lasting Change

In this chapter, we have explored the transformative role that self-care and mindfulness play in the daily management of BPD. By cultivating a routine that honors your physical, mental, and emotional needs, you create a stable foundation from which to navigate life's challenges. The practices discussed—from mindful breathing and body scans to journaling and grounding techniques—are not merely coping mechanisms; they are tools for building resilience, reclaiming your identity, and nurturing your recovery.

Drawing on insights from influential works such as *The Buddha and the Borderline*, *Women Who Run with the Wolves*, *Stop Walking on Eggshells*, and *I Hate You, Don't Leave Me*, we have seen that self-care is both a personal commitment and a radical act of self-love. It empowers you to reclaim your narrative, manage intense emotions, and build a life that is both balanced and fulfilling.

As you continue on your journey, remember that every mindful moment, every act of self-care, and every pause to reflect contributes to your overall well-being. Embrace the process with patience and compassion, knowing that each small step is a victory in itself.

In the next chapter, we will shift our focus to empowerment, resilience, and redefining identity—a deep dive into how the challenges of BPD can be transformed into opportunities for personal growth and self-discovery. With the solid foundation of self-care and mindfulness behind you, you will be even better equipped to embrace the journey ahead, turning vulnerability into strength and chaos into a canvas for renewal.

By integrating clinical insights, practical exercises, and the wisdom of seminal texts, this chapter provides a comprehensive exploration of self-care and mindfulness as vital tools for managing BPD. These practices are not just about surviving each day—they are about thriving, reclaiming your authentic self, and building a future defined by resilience, balance, and self-compassion.

11

Empowerment, Resilience, and Redefining Identity

Empowerment and resilience are not merely abstract ideals; they are the hard-won byproducts of a long and often tumultuous journey through the challenges of Borderline Personality Disorder (BPD). This chapter delves into how women can reclaim their power, foster resilience, and redefine their identity in the wake of emotional upheaval. Drawing on clinical insights, personal narratives, and wisdom from influential texts such as *Women Who Run with the Wolves* by Clarissa Pinkola Estés, *I Hate You, Don't Leave Me* by Jerold J. Kreisman and Hal Straus, *Stop Walking on Eggshells* by Paul Mason and Randi Kreger, and *The Buddha and the Borderline* by Kiera Van Gelder, we will explore practical strategies and reflective practices to empower yourself, nurture resilience, and reconstruct your self-identity.

The Quest for Empowerment

Understanding Empowerment in the Context of BPD

Empowerment, for many women with BPD, means reclaiming control over their emotional lives and redefining themselves beyond the labels imposed by the disorder. It is about recognizing that, despite past traumas and ongoing challenges, you possess the inherent strength to shape your own destiny. In *Women Who Run with the Wolves*, Clarissa Pinkola Estés illustrates how reconnecting with the wild, untamed parts of the feminine spirit can lead to profound self-empowerment. This process involves breaking free from societal constraints and internalized criticisms to embrace a more authentic and vigorous identity.

For those living with BPD, the path to empowerment often begins with accepting vulnerability. As counterintuitive as it may seem, allowing yourself to be vulnerable can be the catalyst for reclaiming your power. Vulnerability opens the door to deep, meaningful connections and enables you to confront and integrate painful experiences rather than letting them define you.

Reframing Negative Narratives

A significant barrier to empowerment is the internal narrative—often harsh and self-critical—that develops over years of emotional turmoil. Books such as *I Hate You, Don't Leave Me* describe how persistent negative self-talk and cognitive distortions can erode self-esteem and reinforce feelings of worthlessness. The journey toward empowerment involves identifying these negative narratives and challenging their validity.

Techniques from Cognitive Behavioral Therapy (CBT) and

Dialectical Behavior Therapy (DBT) can be invaluable in this process. For example, when a negative thought arises—such as "I'm unlovable" or "I always mess things up"—try to reframe it by considering evidence to the contrary. Ask yourself, "What are some moments where I have succeeded or shown love and care?" This practice of cognitive restructuring gradually weakens the hold of negative self-beliefs and paves the way for a more balanced, empowering view of yourself.

Celebrating Small Victories

Empowerment is built gradually, one small victory at a time. Whether it's successfully managing a moment of intense emotion or setting and enforcing a healthy boundary, each success contributes to a growing sense of self-efficacy. In *Stop Walking on Eggshells*, Mason and Kreger emphasize the importance of acknowledging progress, no matter how incremental it may seem. Celebrating these victories reinforces the belief that you are capable of change, and over time, these moments accumulate into a robust sense of empowerment.

Cultivating Resilience

What Is Resilience?

Resilience is the ability to bounce back from setbacks, adapt to adversity, and continue moving forward in the face of challenges. For many with BPD, resilience is not innate but something that must be actively cultivated. It involves developing strategies to manage stress, maintain emotional balance, and recover from crises. Resilience does not mean the absence of pain or difficulty—it means having the strength to persevere despite them.

The transformative power of mindfulness, as explored in *The Buddha and the Borderline*, plays a key role in building resilience. Mindfulness techniques allow you to observe your emotions without judgment, creating the mental space to respond rather than react impulsively. Over time, this practice strengthens your capacity to weather emotional storms, reinforcing the belief that you can survive—and even thrive—despite adversity.

Building Resilience Through Self-Compassion

A core element of resilience is self-compassion—the practice of treating yourself with the same kindness and understanding that you would offer a close friend. Self-compassion is especially important for individuals with BPD, who often face intense self-criticism and shame. By learning to be gentle with yourself, you create an internal support system that nurtures recovery and growth.

In *Women Who Run with the Wolves*, Estés writes about the importance of reconnecting with your instinctual, authentic self—one that is capable of healing and renewal. Self-compassion is the first step in this reconnection. When you allow yourself to experience compassion, you validate your emotions and open up space for healing. This nurturing self-relationship is critical for building resilience, as it reinforces the belief that you are worthy of care and capable of overcoming challenges.

Strategies for Enhancing Resilience

1. **Mindfulness Meditation:**
2. Regular mindfulness practice can help you become more aware of your emotional triggers and develop a calmer response to stress. Techniques such as mindful breathing and body scan meditations provide immediate relief from overwhelming emotions and build long-term emotional resilience.
3. **Journaling:**
4. Keeping a daily journal to track your emotions, successes, and setbacks can offer valuable insights into your resilience journey. Reflecting on your progress allows you to see patterns in your responses and recognize the progress you have made, even during difficult times.
5. **Physical Activity:**
6. Exercise has been shown to reduce stress, improve mood, and enhance overall well-being. Whether it's yoga, walking, or dancing, engaging in physical activity helps release tension and fosters a sense of accomplishment.
7. **Engaging in Creative Outlets:**
8. Creative expression—through art, music, writing, or other forms—can serve as a powerful outlet for processing emotions and building resilience. These activities allow you to externalize your inner experiences and transform them into something beautiful and meaningful.
9. **Social Connection:**
10. Building and maintaining a supportive network is vital for resilience. As discussed in previous chapters, healthy relationships provide emotional support, practical help, and a sense of belonging. Connecting with others who

understand your struggles reinforces your resilience and reminds you that you are not alone.

Redefining Identity

The Crisis of Identity in BPD

One of the most challenging aspects of BPD is the instability of self-identity. Many women with BPD experience a profound crisis of identity, where fluctuating emotions and external pressures make it difficult to form a consistent sense of self. This identity disturbance is not merely a symptom of the disorder—it is a central challenge that affects relationships, decision-making, and overall well-being.

In *I Hate You, Don't Leave Me*, the authors describe how the instability of self-image can lead to a cycle of idealization and devaluation in relationships. Without a stable sense of who you are, it becomes challenging to set boundaries, pursue goals, or even make simple decisions. The journey toward redefining identity is, therefore, both a therapeutic and personal quest— one that requires patience, self-reflection, and a willingness to embrace all facets of your being.

Embracing Complexity and Authenticity

Redefining your identity means acknowledging that you are a multifaceted individual with a complex history—one that includes pain, strength, vulnerability, and beauty. Rather than trying to conform to a single, rigid self-image, consider embracing the full spectrum of your experiences. Your identity is not defined solely by the challenges you face; it is also shaped by your triumphs, your passions, and your unique perspective on the world.

Clarissa Pinkola Estés' *Women Who Run with the Wolves* encourages women to reclaim their wild, authentic selves—a self that has often been suppressed by societal expectations and internalized criticism. Reconnecting with this authentic self involves challenging the limiting beliefs that have been imposed on you and exploring new ways to express your individuality. It is a process of liberation—freeing yourself from the narratives that no longer serve you and constructing an identity that reflects your true nature.

Practical Steps to Redefining Your Identity

1. **Self-Reflection and Exploration:**
2. Take time to explore your interests, values, and passions. Reflect on the experiences that have shaped you and consider how they contribute to your unique identity. Journaling, meditation, and creative pursuits can facilitate this exploration.
3. **Challenging Limiting Beliefs:**
4. Identify the negative beliefs you hold about yourself—such as "I'm unworthy" or "I'm broken"—and actively work to replace them with more balanced, affirming thoughts. Cognitive restructuring techniques from CBT can be particularly helpful in this regard.
5. **Experimenting with New Roles:**
6. Allow yourself the freedom to experiment with different aspects of your personality. Whether it's taking up a new hobby, pursuing a passion project, or engaging in activities that push you out of your comfort zone, these experiences

can help you discover new facets of your identity.

7. **Creating a Personal Narrative:**
8. Construct a narrative that weaves together your past experiences, present challenges, and future aspirations. Narrative therapy techniques can be a powerful tool in this process, helping you to see your life as a story of growth and transformation rather than one of defeat.
9. **Seeking Role Models and Mentors:**
10. Look for individuals—whether in your personal life or through literature and media—who embody the qualities you aspire to develop. Learning from their experiences and perspectives can provide inspiration and practical guidance on redefining your own identity.

Integrating Empowerment, Resilience, and Identity Redefinition

The Interconnected Nature of the Journey

Empowerment, resilience, and identity are deeply interconnected. As you cultivate resilience through mindfulness, self-care, and social support, you gradually build the strength needed to challenge negative narratives and redefine who you are. Every small act of self-compassion or boundary-setting reinforces your sense of empowerment, paving the way for a more coherent and authentic identity.

This integrated process is a dynamic, ongoing journey. There will be moments when setbacks seem to unravel the progress you've made. However, each challenge also provides an opportunity to practice resilience and to refine your understanding of yourself. Over time, you learn that empowerment is not a fixed state—it is a continual process of growth and reinvention.

The Role of Therapeutic Support

Therapy remains a vital component of this journey. Through individual and group therapy sessions, you can gain insights into your emotional patterns, receive guidance on challenging cognitive distortions, and learn strategies to rebuild your self-identity. Resources such as *Stop Walking on Eggshells* offer practical advice on managing interpersonal dynamics, while *The Buddha and the Borderline* provides a compassionate framework for integrating mindfulness into your daily life. Together, these approaches create a robust support system that nurtures empowerment and resilience.

Real-Life Transformations

Countless women have walked this path before you and emerged stronger and more self-assured. Their stories—detailed in personal narratives and clinical case studies—serve as powerful reminders that transformation is possible. Whether it is through overcoming the weight of negative self-talk, learning to trust in one's own strength, or embracing the fullness of one's identity, each journey is a testament to the human capacity for renewal. These real-life examples, found in the pages of works like *I Hate You, Don't Leave Me* and *Women Who Run with the Wolves*, inspire hope and offer practical blueprints for your own journey.

Conclusion: A Future of Possibility

In redefining your identity, embracing empowerment, and cultivating resilience, you lay the foundation for a future defined not by the limitations of BPD but by the possibilities of your true self. This chapter has explored the multifaceted process of reclaiming your power and reconstructing your identity— transforming the challenges of the past into stepping stones for a more authentic and fulfilling future.

By integrating the insights of influential texts, therapeutic practices, and personal experiences, you are invited to see yourself as a dynamic, evolving individual. Every moment of self-compassion, every challenge met with resilience, and every small victory in redefining your identity contributes to a narrative of empowerment. Remember that this journey is ongoing, and each day brings new opportunities to build on the progress you have made.

As you continue forward, keep in mind that the strength you discover within yourself is the catalyst for lasting change. Empowerment is not about denying the pain of the past—it is about transforming that pain into wisdom and using it as fuel for growth. Resilience is not about avoiding adversity; it is about learning how to rise again, stronger and more determined, every time you face a setback.

With the practical strategies and insights shared in this chapter, you now have a roadmap for reclaiming your narrative. Whether it is through mindfulness practices, cognitive reframing, or the courageous act of embracing vulnerability, each step you take is a declaration of your worth and a testament to your enduring strength.

In the next chapter, we will look toward the future by exploring emerging therapies, advocacy efforts, and how you can contribute to a broader conversation about BPD. The empowerment you build today will not only transform your life but can also serve as a beacon of hope for others navigating similar challenges.

By weaving together clinical research, personal narratives, and the timeless wisdom of works such as *Women Who Run with the Wolves*, *I Hate You, Don't Leave Me*, *Stop Walking on Eggshells*, and *The Buddha and the Borderline*, this chapter has offered an in-depth exploration of empowerment, resilience, and identity redefinition. Your journey is a mosaic of pain, strength, transformation, and endless possibility. Embrace every part of it, knowing that each experience contributes to the rich tapestry of who you are and who you are becoming.

Every moment of self-discovery is a victory, and with each step, you empower not only yourself but also inspire others to find their own paths toward healing and authenticity. May this chapter serve as a reminder that no matter how dark the past, the future holds the promise of renewal and boundless potential.

12

Looking Forward – Future Directions in BPD Research and Management

As we reach the final chapter of this book, our focus shifts toward the future—both in terms of research and practical management strategies for Borderline Personality Disorder (BPD). The journey through understanding, treatment, and personal transformation has illuminated many pathways for healing. Now, we turn our attention to emerging therapies, innovative research, advocacy, and policy efforts that promise to redefine the landscape of BPD management. Drawing on insights from seminal texts such as *I Hate You, Don't Leave Me* by Jerold J. Kreisman and Hal Straus, *Stop Walking on Eggshells* by Paul Mason and Randi Kreger, *Women Who Run with the Wolves* by Clarissa Pinkola Estés, and *The Buddha and the Borderline* by Kiera Van Gelder, this chapter offers a comprehensive look at where the field is headed and how these advancements might shape the lives of those affected by BPD.

Emerging Therapeutic Approaches

Innovative Psychotherapies

While Dialectical Behavior Therapy (DBT) and Cognitive Behavioral Therapy (CBT) have long been the mainstays of BPD treatment, the future of psychotherapy for BPD is evolving to address the complexities of the disorder more holistically. Researchers and clinicians are increasingly exploring integrative approaches that blend elements from various therapeutic models.

For instance, **Schema Therapy** is gaining attention as an approach that not only targets negative thought patterns but also addresses the deeper, entrenched schemas that stem from early maladaptive experiences. Schema Therapy helps patients reframe their core beliefs about themselves, fostering a more compassionate self-view. This approach, discussed in extensions of the work presented in *Stop Walking on Eggshells*, offers hope for lasting change by targeting the underlying vulnerabilities of BPD.

Similarly, **Mentalization-Based Treatment (MBT)** focuses on improving the ability to understand the mental states of oneself and others. This therapy is particularly effective in addressing the interpersonal difficulties that are central to BPD, as it trains individuals to interpret social interactions more accurately and empathetically. As research continues to validate MBT, it represents a promising avenue for those struggling with relational instability.

Technological Advances in Therapy

The rapid growth of digital health technologies is reshaping mental health treatment, and BPD is no exception. **Teletherapy** has already expanded access to care for many who might otherwise struggle to attend in-person sessions. Beyond traditional video consultations, emerging digital platforms now offer interactive modules for mindfulness, DBT skills training, and even virtual support groups. These tools provide continuous access to therapeutic resources, which can be especially beneficial during crises or for individuals living in remote areas.

Mobile applications and wearable devices that monitor physiological indicators (such as heart rate variability) are also being integrated into treatment plans. These technologies can alert individuals and their clinicians to early signs of emotional dysregulation, enabling preemptive interventions. As highlighted in *The Buddha and the Borderline*, the intersection of technology and mindfulness offers innovative strategies to ground oneself and regulate emotions in real time.

Pharmacological Innovations

Although no medication has been approved specifically for BPD, ongoing research in psychopharmacology continues to explore options that may address core symptoms more effectively. Researchers are investigating drugs that target specific neurotransmitter systems implicated in emotional regulation and impulse control. For example, advances in understanding the role of serotonin and dopamine in BPD could lead to more targeted treatments with fewer side effects.

Future medication protocols may also incorporate personalized medicine approaches, using genetic and neuroimaging data to tailor treatments to individual neurobiological profiles. Such precision medicine could revolutionize how clinicians approach symptom management, ensuring that pharmacotherapy is both effective and minimally disruptive to patients' lives.

The Role of Neuroscience and Genetics

Advancements in Neuroimaging

Recent advances in neuroimaging techniques are providing unprecedented insights into the brain's structure and function in individuals with BPD. Functional Magnetic Resonance Imaging (fMRI) and Positron Emission Tomography (PET) scans have already revealed patterns of hyperactivity in the amygdala and underactivity in the prefrontal cortex—findings that help explain the emotional volatility and impulsivity seen in BPD.

Future research is likely to build on these findings by mapping the brain's response to various therapeutic interventions. For instance, studies may track changes in neural activity before and after DBT, Schema Therapy, or mindfulness training, providing concrete evidence of how these therapies rewire the brain. Such research not only validates current treatment modalities but also guides the development of new interventions aimed at optimizing brain function and emotional regulation.

Genetics and Epigenetics

In addition to neuroimaging, genetics and epigenetics are emerging as critical areas of investigation. While BPD is influenced by a complex interplay of genetic and environmental factors, identifying specific genetic markers may help predict vulnerability to the disorder. Researchers are exploring how epigenetic modifications—changes in gene expression triggered by environmental factors like trauma—contribute to the development and progression of BPD.

This line of research holds the promise of early identification and intervention. With better genetic screening, it might become possible to recognize at-risk individuals long before the full onset of BPD symptoms, allowing for preventive strategies and early therapeutic engagement. Such advancements could radically shift the paradigm from treatment to prevention, offering hope for reducing the long-term impact of BPD.

Advocacy, Policy, and Public Awareness

Reducing Stigma Through Education

Stigma remains one of the most significant barriers to effective treatment for BPD. Misconceptions about the disorder not only isolate those who suffer from it but also discourage many from seeking help. As detailed in *I Hate You, Don't Leave Me*, societal misunderstandings contribute to a cycle of judgment and exclusion that can worsen the symptoms of BPD.

Future efforts in advocacy will focus on public education campaigns to demystify BPD and highlight its neurobiological and psychosocial underpinnings. By disseminating accurate, research-based information, advocacy groups aim to shift public perceptions from seeing BPD as a character flaw to understanding it as a complex mental health condition. Partnerships between mental health organizations, policymakers, and community leaders are essential in this endeavor, fostering an environment of acceptance and support.

Policy Reforms and Healthcare Access

Effective management of BPD requires comprehensive health-care policies that ensure access to quality treatment. This includes not only mental health services but also community support and crisis intervention resources. Advocacy groups are increasingly calling for policy reforms that integrate mental health care into primary care settings, reducing the fragmenta-tion that often hinders treatment.

Insurance coverage for evidence-based therapies such as DBT, MBT, and Schema Therapy is another critical area of focus. As research continues to demonstrate the efficacy of these interventions, it is imperative that healthcare systems adapt to provide sustained, accessible care for individuals with BPD. Future policy efforts will likely emphasize the importance of long-term support, recognizing that recovery is a gradual, ongoing process rather than a short-term fix.

The Role of Peer Support and Lived Experience

An emerging trend in advocacy is the empowerment of indi-viduals with lived experience. Peer support programs—where individuals who have successfully managed their BPD provide mentorship and guidance—are becoming integral components of mental health services. These programs not only offer prac-tical advice and emotional support but also serve as powerful testimonials to the possibility of recovery.

Public awareness campaigns that feature stories of resilience and transformation can inspire hope and reduce the isolation often experienced by those with BPD. As highlighted in *Women Who Run with the Wolves*, reclaiming one's identity and celebrating the journey toward healing can have a profound impact on public perceptions. Empowering those with BPD to share their stories is a critical step in building a more inclusive, supportive community.

Future Research Directions

Holistic and Integrative Models

The future of BPD research lies in holistic, integrative models that combine biological, psychological, and social perspectives. This comprehensive approach recognizes that BPD is not a monolithic disorder but a dynamic interplay of multiple factors. Researchers are increasingly advocating for studies that examine the interactions between neurobiology, genetics, environmental influences, and therapeutic outcomes.

For example, longitudinal studies that track individuals from early childhood through adulthood can provide invaluable insights into how early trauma and attachment patterns influence the development of BPD. Such research can inform both preventive strategies and the customization of treatment protocols based on individual developmental trajectories.

Innovations in Treatment Delivery

Another promising area of research is the development of novel methods for delivering therapy. Virtual reality (VR) and augmented reality (AR) technologies, for instance, are being explored as tools for creating immersive therapeutic environments. These technologies have the potential to simulate social interactions and trigger emotional responses in controlled settings, providing patients with safe spaces to practice new skills and strategies.

Digital therapeutics, including mobile applications and online platforms, are also poised to revolutionize treatment delivery. These tools can offer real-time support, interactive DBT modules, and access to global peer networks, ensuring that help is always within reach. As these technologies mature, they will likely become standard components of comprehensive BPD management programs.

Personalized Medicine and Biomarkers

The quest for personalized medicine is another frontier in BPD research. By identifying biomarkers—biological indicators that can predict treatment response—clinicians may be able to tailor interventions to individual patients more precisely. This approach could minimize the trial-and-error process currently inherent in psychiatric treatment, leading to faster, more effective outcomes.

Future studies may leverage artificial intelligence (AI) and machine learning to analyze vast datasets, uncovering patterns and predictors of treatment success. The integration of these advanced technologies promises to usher in an era of truly personalized care, where treatments are customized based on a person's unique genetic, neurobiological, and psychosocial profile.

Conclusion: A Vision for the Future

As we look to the future, the management of Borderline Personality Disorder is set to become more precise, holistic, and compassionate. The advances in psychotherapeutic techniques, neuroimaging, genetics, and digital health technologies offer a promising outlook—one where treatment is not only more effective but also more accessible and personalized.

At the heart of this future is the recognition that BPD is a multifaceted condition requiring a multifaceted response. The integration of emerging therapies with established practices, the empowerment of individuals through advocacy and peer support, and the pursuit of research that bridges biology and experience all point toward a new era in BPD management.

As you reflect on the journey detailed in this book—from personal narratives to clinical research and practical strategies—remember that each step forward is a victory. The insights gleaned from works like *I Hate You, Don't Leave Me*, *Stop Walking on Eggshells*, *Women Who Run with the Wolves*, and *The Buddha and the Borderline* remind us that while the challenges of BPD are significant, the potential for healing and growth is even greater.

This vision for the future is one where those affected by BPD are not defined by their struggles but empowered by the knowledge that recovery is possible, that their voices matter, and that they can contribute to a broader conversation about mental health. Through ongoing research, innovative treatment approaches, and compassionate advocacy, we move closer to a world where the stigma surrounding BPD is replaced by understanding, and where every individual has the support needed to thrive.

In closing, the future of BPD research and management is a

collective endeavor—one that calls on clinicians, researchers, policymakers, and, most importantly, individuals with lived experience to join together. Your journey, with all its challenges and triumphs, is a beacon of hope for others. May the insights and tools presented in this book inspire you to embrace your potential, advocate for your well-being, and contribute to the evolving narrative of BPD recovery.

By weaving together the latest scientific research, emerging therapeutic innovations, and the enduring wisdom of seminal texts, this chapter has provided a comprehensive overview of the future directions in BPD research and management. The road ahead is one of promise and possibility—a journey where every new discovery brings us closer to understanding, treating, and ultimately overcoming the challenges of BPD. Embrace the future with optimism, knowing that with each step, you are not only reclaiming your own narrative but also paving the way for a more compassionate and informed approach to mental health for generations to come.